DIGITAL CONTACT TRACING FOR PANDEMIC RESPONSE

DIGITAL CONTACT TRACING FOR PANDEMIC RESPONSE

Ethics and Governance Guidance

Edited by Jeffrey P. Kahn, PhD, MPH, Chair

**Johns Hopkins Project on Ethics and
Governance of Digital Contact Tracing Technologies**

Johns Hopkins University Press

Baltimore

9 8 7 6 5 4 3 2 1

Johns Hopkins University Press
2715 North Charles Street
Baltimore, Maryland 21218-4363
www.press.jhu.edu

Library of Congress Cataloging-in-Publication Data is available.

ISBN 978-1-4214-4061-3 (paperback : acid-free paper)
ISBN 978-1-4214-4062-0 (ebook)
ISBN 978-1-4214-4063-7 (ebook open access)

*Special discounts are available for bulk purchases of this book. For more information,
please contact Special Sales at specialsales@press.jhu.edu.*

Johns Hopkins University Press uses environmentally friendly book materials,
including recycled text paper that is composed of at least 30 percent post-
consumer waste, whenever possible.

Contents

3. Ethics of Designing and Using DCTT 43

4 Legal Considerations 75

5. Recommendations 97

Lead Authors and Contributors

Lead Authors

Joseph Ali, JD. Assistant Professor, Department of International Health, Johns Hopkins Bloomberg School of Public Health; Core Faculty & Associate Director for Global Programs, Johns Hopkins Berman Institute of Bioethics

Anne Barnhill, PhD. Core Faculty & Research Scholar, Johns Hopkins Berman Institute of Bioethics

Anita Cicero, JD. Deputy Director, Johns Hopkins Center for Health Security; Visiting Faculty, Johns Hopkins Bloomberg School of Public Health

Katelyn Esmonde, PhD. Hecht-Levi Postdoctoral Fellow, Johns Hopkins Berman Institute of Bioethics

Amelia Hood, MA. Research Program Coordinator, Johns Hopkins Berman Institute of Bioethics

Brian Hutler, PhD, JD. Hecht-Levi Postdoctoral Fellow, Johns Hopkins Berman Institute of Bioethics

Jeffrey Kahn, PhD, MPH. Andreas C. Dracopoulos Director, Johns Hopkins Berman Institute of Bioethics

Alan Regenberg, MBE. Director of Outreach & Research Support, Associate Faculty, Johns Hopkins Berman Institute of Bioethics

Crystal Watson, DrPH, MPH. Senior Scholar, Johns Hopkins Center for Health Security; Assistant Professor, Department of Environmental Health and Engineering, Johns Hopkins Bloomberg School of Public Health

Matthew Watson. Senior Analyst, Johns Hopkins Center for Health Security; Senior Research Associate, Department of Environmental Health and Engineering, Johns Hopkins Bloomberg School of Public Health

Other Contributors

Robert Califf, MD, MACC. Head of Clinical Policy and Strategy, Verily and Google Health

Ruth Faden PhD, MPH. Philip Franklin Wagley Professor of Biomedical Ethics & Founder, Johns Hopkins Berman Institute of Bioethics

Divya Hosangadi, MSPH. Senior Analyst, Johns Hopkins Center for Health Security; Research Associate, Department of Environmental Health and Engineering, Johns Hopkins Bloomberg School of Public Health

Nancy Kass, ScD. Deputy Director for Public Health & Phoebe R. Berman Professor of Bioethics and Public Health, Johns Hopkins Berman Institute of Bioethics

Alain Labrique, PhD, MHS, MS. Professor, Department of International Health, Johns Hopkins Bloomberg School of Public Health; Director, Johns Hopkins Global Health Initiative

Deven McGraw, JD, MPH, LLM. Chief Regulatory Officer, Ciitizen

Michelle Mello, JD, PhD. Professor of Law, Stanford Law School; Professor of Health Research and Policy, Stanford University School of Medicine

Michael Parker, BEd (Hons), MA, PhD. Director, Wellcome Centre for Ethics and Humanities, Ethox Centre, University of Oxford

Stephen Ruckman, JD, MSc, MAR. Senior Advisor to the President for Policy, Office of the President, Johns Hopkins University

Lainie Rutkow, JD, MPH, PhD. Senior Advisor to the President for National Capital Academic Strategy, Office of the President, Johns Hopkins University

Josh Sharfstein, MD. Vice Dean for Public Health Practice and Community Engagement, Professor of the Practice, Johns Hopkins Bloomberg School of Public Health

Jeremy Sugarman, MD, MPH, MA. Deputy Director for Medicine, Harvey M. Meyerhoff Professor of Bioethics and Medicine, Johns Hopkins Berman Institute of Bioethics; Department of Medicine, Johns Hopkins School of Medicine; and Department of Health Policy and Management, Johns Hopkins Bloomberg School of Public Health

Eric Toner, MD. Senior Scholar, Johns Hopkins Center for Health Security; Senior Scientist, Department of Environmental Health and Engineering, Johns Hopkins Bloomberg School of Public Health

Marc Trotochaud, MSPH. Analyst, Johns Hopkins Center for Health Security; Research Associate, Department of Environmental Health and Engineering, Johns Hopkins Bloomberg School of Public Health

Effy Vayena, PhD. Professor, Health Ethics & Policy Lab, Department of Health Sciences & Technology, ETH Zurich

Tal Zarsky, JSD, LLM, LLB. Professor of Law, University of Haifa Faculty of Law; Visiting Scholar, University of Pennsylvania Law School (2019–2020)

Preface

Digital technologies are being developed and promoted to support the public health response to the COVID-19 pandemic, with discussion and implementation planning in the United States by localities, states, institutions, and employers. Key decision makers and stakeholders—including government officials, institutional leaders, employers, digital technology developers, and the public—require clear and well-supported guidance to inform the deployment and use of these technologies as well as of the data they collect, store, and share. While technology-based approaches are currently unable to provide solutions on their own, experiences in other countries indicate that they could be used successfully in conjunction with traditional and novel public health methods.

This report reflects a rapid research and expert consensus group effort led by the Berman Institute of Bioethics and the Center for Health Security at Johns Hopkins University. It draws on experts from both inside and outside Johns Hopkins in bioethics, health security, public health, technology development, engineering, public policy, and law. The report highlights issues that must be addressed and provides recommendations for the use of digital technologies as part of contact tracing.

The analysis offered here is focused on answering the following questions:

- Can digital contact tracing technologies (DCTT) be effective as part of public health responses to the pandemic, and if so, to what degree, for which specific types of functions, with what confidence, and with what requirements?

- How can these technologies serve the interests of public health while respecting other individual and collective interests, such as ensuring equitable distribution of benefits and burdens and limiting infringement on privacy and other civil liberties?

- What are the ethical, legal, policy, and governance guardrails currently in place around such technologies and what else is needed?
- What additional guardrails are required to ensure that the goals of public health in using these technologies are achievable in ways that are ethically and legally sound?

To answer these questions, the report examines some core aspects of digital technologies applied to contact tracing, focusing on:

- the value of and basic methods for traditional public health surveillance and contact tracing,
- candidate technological products to enhance public health surveillance and contact tracing, how they work, and their comparative value for public health,
- core ethical, legal, and governance considerations, and how they relate to relevant features of candidate technological solutions, and
- what is needed to move forward responsibly with the use of digital technology in support of public health surveillance, acknowledging gaps in our current understanding.

The project involved in-depth analysis by a dedicated team of faculty, postdoctoral fellows, and research staff working over the course of only a few weeks but with great intensity, drafting a report in collaboration with 26 total contributors writing, commenting, and revising through multiple drafts, with the penultimate draft "pressure-tested" by review and discussion at a virtual workshop of invited experts and stakeholders held on May 13, 2020, and the final version completed on May 21, 2020. The report and analysis builds on the excellent work of others in some parts of this territory, while focusing on the gaps in analysis and areas that have not been sufficiently addressed. The goal is to offer comprehensive guidance to relevant stakeholders to advance public health response during the COVID-19 pandemic. Given the rapidly evolving territory into which DCTT is being introduced, this report will, by necessity, be something of a living document, updated as often as information dictates in order to continue to offer leading-edge analysis and guidance. Versions will be noted in the digital and print editions.

Acknowledgments

Efforts like this project require teams and even small armies to be carried out successfully, and this was no exception, except that it was many fewer people working many more hours than could reasonably be expected of them. From the initial kernel of an idea to the publication of this report in book form, this project took just over a month total. That seems impossible, even as I know it is accurate, and it speaks to the incredible commitment, hard work, research skills, and analytic acumen of our colleagues at Johns Hopkins—the core team are deservedly listed as lead authors of this report.

None of this would have been possible without the support—moral and financial—and encouragement of Johns Hopkins University President Ronald J. Daniels, who was the first to suggest the idea to me of taking on this topic. He provided not only support and encouragement but the imprimatur of his office, including help, guidance, and counsel from Prof. Lainie Rutkow, senior advisor to the president. Lainie played a more integral role than that description captures, reflected in part by her inclusion among the report's contributors, but she deserves special acknowledgement for shepherding us through to the end.

I mentioned that this was a team effort, and every team requires an effective leader. My colleague Prof. Joseph Ali stepped into that role as we undertook the project, and then he worked seven days a week along with the rest of the core research and writing team, always unfailingly positive and deeply engaged in the work. He, along with Prof. Anne Barnhill, Alan Regenberg, Amelia Hood, and Drs. Katelyn Esmonde, Brian Hutler, and Crystal Watson, all deserve special thanks for doing so much in so little time, all while working under the grinding social distancing restrictions of the 2020 pandemic. That work was supported by Arnold & Porter Kaye Scholer LLP with legal research and other assistance—a huge thanks to them. Finally, the 16 contributing authors were incredibly generous with their time, energy, and insights, all on ridiculously tight timelines, and never a complaint or objection.

The project benefited greatly from a number of experts who provided written feedback on drafts and who attended the virtual workshop to test our recommendations, including Miles Stewart, Rob Nichols, Smisha Aagarwal, Karl Steiner, Anupam Joshi, Charles Scheeler, Ford Rowan, and Jay Wagley.

Last, the fact that this report appears in published book form by Johns Hopkins University Press is another minor miracle, from manuscript to printed book in under a week. Thanks to JHUP Director Barbara Kline Pope and her team for being willing to take on the challenge and for the incredible focused effort it required.

MY HEARTFELT THANKS AND
APPRECIATION TO YOU ALL,

Jeffrey Kahn

Acronyms and Abbreviations

ADA   Americans with Disabilities Act
BLE   Bluetooth Low Energy
CalOPPA   California Online Privacy Protection Act
CBP   Customs and Border Protection
CCPA   California Consumer Privacy Act
CDC   Centers for Disease Control and Prevention
CLOUD Act   Clarifying Lawful Overseas Use of Data Act
COPPA   Children's Online Privacy Protection Act
COV+   confirmed positive SARS-CoV-2 test result
COVID-19   coronavirus disease 2019
CPNI   customer proprietary network information
CSLI   cell-site location information
DCTT   digital contact tracing technology and closely related
                digital health products
ECPA   Electronic Communications Privacy Act
EEOC   Equal Employment Opportunity Commission
E-SIGN   Electronic Signatures in Global and National
                Commerce Act
EU   European Union
FCC   Federal Communications Commission
FTC   Federal Trade Commission
FTCA   Federal Trade Commission Act
GIS   geographic information system
GPS   global positioning system
HHS   US Department of Health and Human Services
HIPAA   Health Insurance Portability and Accountability Act
HIV   human immunodeficiency virus
ICU   intensive care unit

IRB	institutional review board
JHU	Johns Hopkins University
OCR	Office for Civil Rights, US Department of Health & Human Services
OSHA	Occupational Safety and Health Administration
PHI	protected health information
PII	personally identifiable information
PPE	personal protective equipment
PPPT	privacy-preserving proximity tracking
QR Code	quick response code
RFRA	Religious Freedom Restoration Act
RLUIPA	Religious Land Use and Institutionalized Persons Act
SARS-CoV-2	severe acute respiratory syndrome coronavirus 2
SCA	Stored Communications Act
STI	sexually transmitted infection

DIGITAL CONTACT TRACING FOR PANDEMIC RESPONSE

Summary

Introduction

Public health professionals around the world are working tirelessly to respond to the COVID-19 pandemic using tried-and-tested public health methods for infectious disease surveillance and control. These traditional methods are essential to the global COVID-19 response. To complement these actions and potentially augment the speed and efficacy of the public health workforce, digital technologies are being harnessed. Given the scale of the pandemic, significant efforts are being undertaken to develop and leverage public-facing and health-system-supportive technology solutions, including smartphone apps and other digital tools, that may aid public health surveillance and contact tracing.

Digital contact tracing technology and closely related digital health products (together DCTT) have been used in several countries as part of broader disease surveillance and containment strategies. In the United States, DCTT has been proposed as an integral part of some plans to "reopen" the country (Allen et al. 2020; Hart et al. 2020; Simpson and Conner 2020). It is almost certain that these and related technologies will become part of not only the COVID-19 response but also the larger toolbox for future public health communicable disease prevention and control.

These technologies have significant promise. They also raise important ethical, legal, and governance challenges that require comprehensive analysis in order to support decision-making. Government officials, public health leaders, leaders of institutions, employers, digital technology developers, and the public all must be adequately informed in order to make

1

responsible choices. Johns Hopkins University recognized the importance of helping to guide this process. It organized an expert group with members from inside and outside of Hopkins and led by its Berman Institute of Bioethics in collaboration with the Center for Health Security. Its charge was to examine the ethics, law, policy, and public health implications of using digital technologies as part of pandemic response and to develop guidance, including a framework and actionable recommendations, for governmental and institutional decision makers.

Overall, this expert group urges a stepwise approach that prioritizes alignment of technology with public health needs and public values, building choice into design architecture, and capturing real-world results and impacts to allow adjustments as required. Further, we urge an approach that recognizes that there are complicated issues to resolve for governments, institutions, and businesses and that introduction of DCTT must include public engagement and ongoing assessments to improve both performance and adoption.

Specific recommendations include the following:

- There is no "one size fits all" approach to DCTT. Technology design should not be static, but it should be capable of evolving depending upon local conditions, new evidence, and changing preferences and priorities.
- Technology companies alone should not control the terms, conditions, or capabilities of DCTT, nor should they presume to know what is acceptable to members of the public.
- DCTT should be designed to have a base set of features that protect privacy, with layers of additional capabilities that users may choose to activate. An initial default should be that user location data are not shared, but users should be provided with easy mechanisms and prompts to allow for opting-in to this capability, with encouragement to the public if it is shown to be critical to achieving public health goals.
- Data collected through DCTT should be made available to public health professionals and to researchers in de-identified form to support population-level epidemiologic analyses.

- Those who authorize use of DCTT within a particular jurisdiction or institution should continuously and systematically monitor the technology's performance in that context. This should include monitoring for effectiveness and benefit, monitoring for harms, and monitoring for the fair distribution of both benefits and harms.
- Governments should not require mandatory use of DCTT given uncertainty about potential burdens and benefits. Additional technology, user, and real-world testing is needed.

Through in-depth analysis and recommendations, this report seeks to guide decision-making and enhance understanding of

- the value of and basic methods for traditional public health surveillance and contact tracing,
- candidate technological products to enhance public health surveillance and contact tracing, and their comparative value for public health,
- core ethical, legal, policy, and governance considerations, and how they relate to relevant features of candidate technological solutions, and
- what is needed to move forward responsibly with the use of digital technology in support of public health surveillance, acknowledging gaps in our current understanding.

The full set of recommendations are intended to (1) support effective and informed adoption of DCTT, (2) encourage design of flexible technologies that maximize public health utility while respecting other values, (3) establish meaningful processes for user disclosure and authorization (consent), (4) promote equity and fairness in the uses of DCTT, and (5) foster transparent governance and oversight.

DCTT Features, Functions, and Potential Applications

Digital contact tracing technologies and platforms can be roughly categorized into three broad approaches along a spectrum of potential policies and methods: a **maximal approach** (typified by the South Korean government's centralized and triangulated data collection (M. S. Kim 2020)); a **minimal approach** (typified by the Apple/Google decentralized privacy-preserving proximity tracking (PPPT) and contact notification (Apple and Google n.d.)); and a diverse range of **middle-ground approaches** that aim to augment manual contact tracing with the collection of digital data that can be shared with public health authorities.

Minimal approaches, such as the Apple/Google PPPT, use Bluetooth Low Energy (BLE) "handshakes" that record close contact between mobile phone users but do not register the location in which the contact happened. In most architectures, these proximity data are stored in the users' phones as anonymized "beacons" that cannot be used to re-identify the users directly. If a user with a PPPT app installed on their phone tests positive and enters test results into their app, those who have been in contact with them can be notified by the app. This "exposure notification" can be automatic or at the discretion of the COV+ person, depending on the app design. If notified, a user who has been in contact with a COV+ individual would receive a push notification alerting them to possible exposure (which may be timestamped), but with no other identifying information.

The most prevalent **middle-ground approach** in the US context involves the collection and storage of personal data—including identifying information and location data—on the user's phone. These decentralized but personally identifiable data can then be voluntarily shared with public health officials if the user tests positive for SARS-CoV-2 (severe acute respiratory syndrome coronavirus 2). For example, a team at the Massachusetts Institute of Technology (MIT) has developed an app called Private Kit: Safe Paths (MIT n.d.) that stores users' location data on their phone for 28 days. If a user tests positive, she can voluntarily upload her location data to a website that is accessible only to public health officials. Officials can then analyze these personally identifiable data and, subsequently, broadcast redacted and de-identified data to other users. Healthy users would have access to these redacted location data of COV+ users, but their own data would not leave their phones. At a minimum, the storage of user location data can function as a "memory aid" if the user tests positive, but releasing the data to public health authorities may help to analyze the spread of SARS-CoV-2 and alert individuals or groups that have been in contact with COV+ patients.

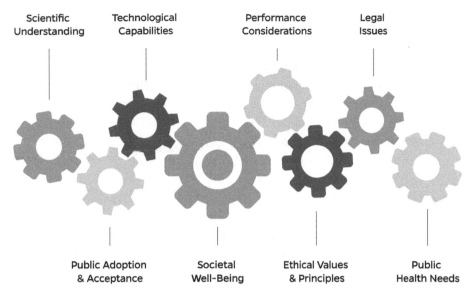

Scientific Understanding Technological Capabilities Performance Considerations Legal Issues

Public Adoption & Acceptance Societal Well-Being Ethical Values & Principles Public Health Needs

FIGURE 1   Interrelating Factors That Frame Responsible Development of Digital Contact Tracing Technology

The US Centers for Disease Control and Prevention (CDC) has published preliminary criteria for evaluating capabilities and attributes of DCTT (CDC 2020e). These and other resources suggest that a comprehensive assessment of DCTT and its potential to advance the public's health will require careful consideration of numerous interconnected factors that interact in complex ways and must be navigated within the challenging contexts of uncertainty and urgent need (Figure 1). These include:

- scientific and epidemiological understanding of SARS-CoV-2 transmission and infection,
- public health needs for combating the outbreak,
- technological capabilities of DCTT,
- performance of DCTT applications,
- ethical values and principles,
- characteristics of public adoption and acceptance, and
- legal issues and landscape.

The primary objectives for use of DCTT during the COVID-19 pandemic must be to reduce illness and death and facilitate public health efforts to reduce transmission of the virus. These objectives fall under a broader overall goal of contributing to societal well-being during the pandemic. It is not yet known whether and how much DCTT can contribute to these primary objectives, nor whether it will be able to contribute without generating new burdens or even harms, such as incorrect warnings or "noise" that detract from the work of manual contact tracing.

The process of identifying acceptable technology designs and uses is complex, given the interplay among the factors. Our analysis reveals that there is no "one size fits all" approach to DCTT. There is variability across the United States with respect to SARS-CoV-2 prevalence and infection rates, public health capacity, public attitudes toward DCTT, and acceptability of various potential features. Moreover, our understanding of SARS-CoV-2 and DCTT is evolving, public health response needs and capabilities are changing, and public attitudes are shifting. Different technologies used in different ways may be appropriate to achieve slightly different public health goals in different localities and at different points in the pandemic. A tiered and phased approach to technology development should be facilitated by law and policy, prioritizing underlying interoperability, while permitting user choices now and for the future.

Given the complexity of the terrain, as a first step, those developing or considering widespread use of DCTT as part of pandemic response should be guided by the following principles and related actions (see box). These principles are meant to apply to DCTT, as well as other digital technologies used in novel ways during pandemic response.

These principles make clear that in order to *maximize* the public good from use of DCTT, public health needs and technological capabilities must be carefully aligned. Government officials, public health leaders, leaders of other institutions, employers, digital technology developers, and the public are all key stakeholders that must be informed and engaged in order to enable the most successful and ethically acceptable uses of DCTT.

Guiding Principles for the Use of Digital Public Health Technologies for Pandemic Response

Transparency and public engagement are essential to an inclusive digital public health response

- Government, public health, and digital technology leaders must engage effectively with the public and other stakeholders to communicate the utility, importance, oversight, and limitations of relevant digital technologies, including their implications for individuals' privacy and civil liberties.
- Transparency at all levels is essential for maintaining public trust and confidence.
- To the extent possible, digital public health responses should reflect the range of values that are important to individuals, including advancing the health and well-being of the community as a whole.
- Decision makers should recognize the sacrifices that some people may be willing to make during a pandemic in order to advance public health goals. Acceptance by some of particular monitoring capabilities should not be read as a willingness to extend these methods to other problems or uses.

Digital public health responses must represent the least infringement of civil liberties necessary to accomplish the public health goals

- If preferred digital public health strategies infringe on privacy and other civil liberties, the infringements must be sufficiently justified by the circumstances of the pandemic, offset by ample anticipated public benefit, and considered relative to infringements associated with other possible strategies, such as mass physical distancing.
- Only those data that are necessary and relevant for the stated public health purposes should be collected. Identifiable data should be stored in a secure manner and only for the period of time that the public health purposes require.
- Adopted technologies should not be used in ways that subject communities to discrimination or surveillance for non–public health reasons.
- Respect for individual autonomy requires that users are sufficiently informed of the public health goals of the technology and the extent to which those goals are being met.

Use of digital public health technologies and data must be guided by best available evidence

- Decisions to deploy digital public health technologies should be based on a careful assessment of the uses and limitations of any proposed technology, taking into account the best available evidence.

- Those who deploy digital public health technologies should continuously and systematically monitor their performance, as well as any evidence that is being generated in other contexts about the selected technological solution and about other competing technologies.
- Unintended consequences—including those that might impact public health goals, core values and interests of the public, and unfair advantage or disadvantage—should be carefully monitored and addressed as necessary.

Responsible use of digital public health technology requires meaningful governance and accountability

- Systems of governance must be trustworthy and well informed. They must be reviewed and adjusted as circumstances and evidence change or as unintended effects are identified.
- Trusted representatives who are capable of developing and implementing uniform and fair standards for adopting and utilizing underlying digital technology must be identified.
- Understandable, transparent, and publicly accessible rules must guide the collection, access, control, use, storage, and combination of data by government authorities, public and private institutions, and other parties such as public health researchers.
- Oversight, accountability, and consequences for abuse or misuse of these data must be explicit and enforceable.

The deployment of digital public health technology must be rooted in a commitment to equity

- Digital public health technologies should be deployed in a manner that does not propagate preexisting patterns of unfair disadvantage or further distribute harms and risks unfairly throughout the population.
- To the extent possible, digital public health technologies should be designed to rectify existing inequities.
- Oversight mechanisms must be in place to ensure that the improved public health outcomes are equitable and to detect and correct any unforeseen resultant injustices attributable to the technology or that can be addressed using the technology.
- The incentives and disincentives for adopting new technology must be equitable, not exploitative, and aligned with effective use of the technology.
- Disparity-driven technology gaps should be explicitly recognized. To the extent possible, provisions should be made to address the digital divide.

Summary of Recommendations

The guidance document makes a number of recommendations related to (1) supporting effective and informed adoption of DCTT, (2) designing flexible technologies to maximize public health utility while respecting other values, (3) establishing meaningful processes for user disclosure and authorization/consent, (4) promoting equity and fairness in application of DCTT, and (5) instituting transparent governance and oversight. Here we provide a summary of recommendations.

Supporting Effective and Informed Adoption

- Those who authorize use of DCTT within a particular jurisdiction or institution should continuously and systematically monitor the technology's performance in that context. This should include monitoring for effectiveness and benefit, monitoring for harms, and monitoring for the fair distribution of both benefits and harms. They should also monitor evidence that is being generated in other contexts about their selected technological solution and about other competing technologies.

- Data collected through DCTT should be made available to public health professionals and to researchers in de-identified form to support population-level epidemiologic analysis.

- Data should be available to users that would permit them to further investigate their personal risk with public health officials or other health workers to add a layer of protection against unnecessary quarantine.

- Technologies or apps may produce some false negatives or false positives, but they should be accurate enough that public health authorities feel confident that they support, and don't detract from, contact tracing efforts.

- Trusted leaders should be enlisted to communicate effectively with the public about DCTT and encourage its use should the technology demonstrate some potential. The limits of knowledge regarding effectiveness should also be explained along with what will be done to improve technological capabilities as understanding evolves.

- Incentives can be a useful complement to encouragements; however, any incentives for users to install and use DCTT must be equitable, should not be coercive, and should align with effective use of the technology.

- DCTT use should not be mandated at this time given uncertainty about potential harms and benefits. Additional technology, user, and real-world testing is needed.

Designing Flexible Technology to Maximize Public Health Utility While Respecting Other Values

- Technology companies should not alone control the terms, conditions, or capabilities of DCTT, nor should they presume to know what is acceptable to members of the public.

- A "values in design" approach to development of DCTT should be adopted (Flanagan, Howe, and Nissenbaum 2008; Knobel and Bowker 2011). Robust public and user engagement activities should be pursued to identify and incorporate, to the extent possible, a range of values into the design of the technology. These values may include privacy, but also autonomy, efficiency, equity, or others. Technology design should reflect an appropriate balance and prioritization of identified values.

- Technology design should not be static, but should be capable of evolving depending upon local conditions, new evidence, and changing preferences and priorities.

- DCTT should be designed to have a base set of features that protect privacy, with layers of additional capabilities that users may choose to activate. An initial default should be that user location data are not shared, but users should be provided with easy mechanisms and prompts to allow for opting-in to this capability, with encouragement to the public if it is shown to be critical to achieving public health goals.

Establishing Meaningful Processes for User Disclosure and Authorization (Consent)

- A clear and concise module consisting of basic disclosure and voluntary authorization should be developed to accompany DCTT.

This module should not take the form of "clickwrap" terms of service or end-user agreements but rather provide only essential information necessary for an individual to make a decision. More detailed disclosures (such as FAQs in plain language) should be made easily accessible to those who wish to learn more, with no hidden surprises.

- An opt-in approach to authorization should be instituted to accompany initial DCTT rollout. The feasibility and value of opt-out approaches should continue to be evaluated, informed by what is technologically possible, what local assessments of benefits and harms of the technology reveal over time, and our evolving understanding of the degree to which an opt-out approach is likely to increase or decrease utilization among different populations. Opt-out approaches should not be precluded.

Promoting Equity and Fairness in Application of DCTT

- States, localities, and institutions that recommend widespread use of DCTT should provide technology (e.g., mobile phones, Bluetooth devices) and free data packages to those who desire but lack access to these devices.
- If there are lower rates of adoption of DCTT systems in some identifiable communities, public health authorities should find ways to compensate. For example, directing more non-DCTT resources and efforts toward those communities to meet specific needs that are elsewhere being supported by technology.
- If maps are generated based on DCTT to provide the public with the locations that COV+ individuals have visited, steps must be taken to minimize the stigma and potential financial losses that could result from a location being identified as a hotspot.

Instituting Transparent Governance and Oversight

- Digital surveillance oversight committees should be established expeditiously, with diverse and qualified membership, to provide ethical and regulatory review prior to and concurrent with widespread use of a DCTT system.
- Understandable and publicly accessible rules must guide the col-

lection, access, control, use, storage, and combination of data by government authorities, public and private institutions, and other parties such as public health researchers.

- Only those data that are necessary and relevant for the public health response to COVID-19 should be collected and used.

- Identifiable data should be kept only for the period of time needed for the public health response to COVID-19.

- Identifiable data collected as part of this response should not be shared with anyone other than the relevant public health authorities without additional specific informed consent of individual users.

- Before a government or institution adopts a digital contact tracing program, they should state the conditions under which the digital contact tracing program will be terminated.

- Future use of DCTT to advance public health or other efforts (e.g., use in seasonal flu surveillance) would require independent justification. DCTT designed for public health use should not be used by law or immigration enforcement.

- The principles offered in this guidance document apply both during and following the COVID-19 pandemic.

Legislative Recommendations

- The United States Congress should enact new legislation, specifically tailored to facilitate the use of DCTT as part of the public health response to COVID-19, while also protecting user privacy and ensuring data security.

- Congress should require DCTT developers to disclose to users, in clear language, the nature of the information that would be collected, how it would be collected, how it would be stored, and for what purposes it may be used.

- While the rollout of DCTT should initially employ an opt-in authorization approach, the feasibility, acceptability, and value of opt-out approaches should continue to be evaluated. As such, opt-out approaches to consent should not be precluded by legislation.

- Congress should prohibit the commercial use of data collected for COVID-19 response by DCTT.

- Congress should prohibit discrimination on the basis of data collected by DCTT.

- If Congress is unable to enact suitable legislation, state legislatures should work toward enacting similar laws for their jurisdictions. A "model" state law should be rapidly developed to facilitate nationwide adoption of an appropriate law and uniformity of legal requirements.

Summary of Analysis

Supporting Effective and Informed Adoption

The COVID-19 pandemic and the physical distancing efforts implemented to slow the rate of transmission have caused severe harm to individuals, communities, and our society. To protect the public good going forward, we need a robust public health response that reduces the spread of SARS-CoV-2 and does so in a way that allows economic recovery to occur and to be sustained. We also need to design and manage this public health response so as to minimize harms to individuals and society, to distribute benefits and burdens equitably across the population, and to avoid misuses of the technologies and the data they collect.

To reduce the spread of SARS-CoV-2, chains of transmission need to be broken. To do this, people who have been exposed to SARS-CoV-2, or potentially exposed, need to be identified as comprehensively and as quickly as possible so they can quarantine themselves and avoid infecting others. This is the job of manual contact tracing by public health authorities, in which people infected or presumptively infected with SARS-CoV-2 are interviewed and asked about their movements and interactions, including where they work and shop, how they travel, with whom they've had contact, and the nature of that contact (e.g., where the contact took place). Their contacts are then interviewed and potentially asked to quarantine, seek testing, and take other protective measures if the contact is sufficiently high risk.

The hope is that DCTT can augment traditional contact tracing efforts, either by working alongside and independently of manual contact tracing or by being integrated into manual contact tracing efforts in a way that makes these efforts faster, more thorough, and more efficient.

Data suggest that a substantial proportion of transmissions—perhaps as high as 50%—occur between individuals who are not symptomatic and that transmission may occur as early as 3 days before onset of symptoms (WHO 2020). Because asymptomatic spread of SARS-CoV-2 appears to be a significant source of infection, we need to identify potentially infected people before they show symptoms; thus, speed is of the essence. This is one benefit of using DCTT: potential contacts can be identified instantaneously, notified quickly, and asked to quarantine as soon as possible.

Another benefit is identifying contacts who manual contact tracing methods may miss, either because COV+ people do not remember all the places they've been or cannot identify all the people they've had contact with. This is especially relevant given the long period of infectivity of SARS-CoV-2, which begins before people are symptomatic and aware they are infected (Ferretti et al. 2020). If DCTT were designed to have optional location-monitoring capabilities, this critical challenge could be mitigated even further. For example, location data might reveal that a COV+ person was at a restaurant at an exact time and date, which could be followed up by contact tracers who could alert the public or use other measures to reach those who were also present in the restaurant at the same time. In other disease contexts, geolocation data have demonstrated some potential to support epidemiology and disease surveillance (see Furlanello et al. 2002; Dredze et al. 2013; Eckhoff and Tatem 2015; Fraccaro et al. 2019), with technical cautions regarding accuracy and the like (Beukenhorst et al. 2017).

One role for DCTT is to work alongside manual contact tracing but independently of it. Individuals would download proximity tracing or exposure notification apps, use them, receive alerts if they've had a potential contact with another user who is COV+ or presumptively COV+, and voluntarily self-quarantine without having contact with public health authorities or giving them data that feeds into public health contact tracing efforts. It is possible that this would help to break chains of transmission and reduce the spread of SARS-CoV-2, though at this point these benefits are speculative. It is also possible that such exposure notifications will result in high rates of false positives.

Another possible role is for DCTT to be integrated into manual contact tracing efforts. When potential contacts are identified by DCTT, they are connected to public health authorities who can then follow up with them. There are different forms this could take and different kinds and amounts of data about contacts public health authorities could receive from DCTT. On one end of the spectrum of reporting, public health authorities would not receive individuals' names or contact information, only anonymous data. The fullest version of reporting would securely send to public health authorities the names, contact information such as address and phone number, and other data about contacts that DCTT collected, including data about their location and movement history.

It is uncertain whether providing public health authorities with volumes of information on cases and contacts from DCTT will be useful in practice. As mentioned above, providing public health authorities with location data on cases and contacts collected by DCTT may help contact tracers to find and notify additional contacts. However, at present, providing public health authorities with large amounts of data will be useful only if there is sufficient capacity to follow up on these data. In addition, there is a risk of low-quality data from DCTT flooding the system, leading to investigation of false case contacts identified by DCTT and distracting from other important efforts. Whether and to what extent data from DCTT will benefit contact tracing efforts is unknown, pointing again to the importance of continuously collecting high-quality evidence about DCTT.

Designing Flexible Technology to Maximize
Public Health Utility While Respecting Other Values

Use of DCTT is essentially an experiment, as we have insufficient information about the performance of different DCTT and their efficacy. In the face of this uncertainty, how should DCTT be designed and how should its use be managed?

Many efforts to advance DCTT in the United States and elsewhere have emphasized the importance of "privacy by design"; that is, building privacy and security protections into the design of technology rather than counting on responsible use alone (Cavoukian 2010). As noted above, some major technology companies have signaled this position through development of PPPT systems that embed features such as decentralization, de-identified information, user anonymity, bans on collection of location data, and minimal reliance on or integration of public health authorities or other government actors. Many of these features have also been embraced early by advocacy organizations (Crocker, Opsahl, and Cyphers 2020; Electronic Privacy Information Center 2020; Kahn Gilmor 2020) and in an open letter ("Joint Statement on Contact Tracing" 2020) from nearly 300 researchers. These same actors have emphasized that use of DCTT should be fully voluntary.

Although privacy is a key value, individuals and communities may also value efficiency, equity, liberty, autonomy, economic well-being, companionship, patriotism, or solidarity, among other values. People may accept more significant encroachments on privacy now if this ultimately results in realizing other values (such as companionship) that are of equal or greater importance to those individuals. Rather than centering privacy alone in design, a different orientation is needed at this moment: that of "values in design," which incorporates a broader range of values into technology (Flanagan, Howe, and Nissenbaum 2008; Knobel and Bowker 2011). For example, some users might wish to express autonomy, solidarity, or patriotism through DCTT by sharing their location history with public health professionals in order to advance the public health response, increase system efficiencies (e.g., by contributing information that can lead to better data processing), and reduce the burden on essential workers. At the same time, there is value in further advancing autonomy by designing technology to allow individuals some control over what data about them are collected and shared.

DCTT should be designed to have a base set of features that protect privacy and strive for interoperability, but also should include other optional capabilities. This could be achieved by designing DCTT to have a default that can be modified: for example, an initial setting could be that users' location data are not shared with public health authorities, but users may opt-in to this feature. Such an opt-in approach is likely consistent with existing federal privacy laws.

Designing DCTT this way gives users the flexibility to decide how to use the technology and how to engage with public health authorities, consistent with their values and trade-offs they are willing to make. This flexibility could also allow for more real-world evaluation of how different users experience different features of DCTT in different locations. Technology design should not be static, but it should be capable of evolving depending upon local conditions, new evidence, and changing preferences and priorities.

DCTT developers must comply with a number of federal privacy laws. These privacy laws generally permit the collection, storage, and use of personal information, so long as the user provides meaningful consent. Privacy law in the United States is generally sector-specific and limited in scope, resulting in a patchwork of protections that differ significantly depending on the entity that collects the data and the type of data collected. Given the complexity of existing federal privacy law and the need to further strengthen public trust in DCTT, it would be beneficial for Congress to enact new privacy legislation that is specifically tailored to the use of DCTT in response to COVID-19. Such COVID-specific legislation should be sensitive to the full range of values and recommendations described above.

In short, designing "middle-ground" DCTT for flexible use may provide the most adaptable and thus most robust public health response—respecting privacy and individual autonomy by allowing users to use DCTT in ways that express their own values.

Public Acceptance of DCTT

While some groups have maintained that only PPPT-like minimal systems will be widely adopted, because only they will earn and maintain public trust (Simpson and Conner 2020), there is insufficient evidence that public trust would be threatened by a DCTT system that has the capacity to securely collect location data, integrate public health authorities, and enable voluntary sharing of certain user data (e.g., location data) with those authorities. More research, including through deliberative engagement sessions, is needed to better understand how differences in the features and functionality of DCTT (such as optional sharing of geolocation data) influence trust and people's willingness to use DCTT. Technology companies should not alone control the terms, conditions, and capabilities of DCTT, nor should they presume to know what is acceptable to members of the public.

Significant concerns have also been expressed by privacy advocates (Guariglia 2020) and in the popular press (Giglio 2020) about "surveillance creep"—that is, a belief that state or corporate actors will use new surveillance technologies, capacities, and permissions well beyond the purposes for which they were initially justified to the public and beyond the time when they are useful for the COVID-19 pandemic. Surveillance creep is a serious concern and should be carefully guarded against; however, the possibility of surveillance creep is not a sufficient reason to limit development of DCTT to minimal systems. Instead, protections should be put in place to ensure that only those data that are necessary and relevant for the public health purposes at hand are collected and used, and data should be kept only for the period of time needed for those public health purposes. For this reason, we would support COVID-specific legislation that would impose strict limits on the use of DCTT data for non–public health purposes.

Finally, the use of DCTT during the current pandemic should not set a precedent for future public health use (e.g., use in seasonal flu surveillance efforts). Future use would require independent justification. Further, use of DCTT in other contexts (e.g., by law enforcement or immigration enforcement) is presumptively unethical.

Encouraging Adoption of DCTT

Researchers have estimated, perhaps conservatively, that DCTT use by 80% of smartphone owners, or 56% of the population overall, will be needed to suppress the epidemic (Hinch et al. 2020). These estimates also highlight that some decrease in transmission would be realizable even with lower rates of technology adoption.

In the United States, many advocates and researchers have argued that use of DCTT must be fully voluntary. However, experience from other countries suggests that when use of a digital contact tracing app is voluntary, only a minority of the population will download it. Instead of making use fully voluntary and initiated by users, there are ways that DCTT could be put into use without users' voluntary choice. For example, use of an app could be mandated as a precondition for returning to work or school, or even further, to control entry into a facility or transportation (such as airplanes) through scanning of a QR code to demonstrate personal exposure levels (Gan and Culver 2020).

While these approaches are hard to imagine in the United States, some have argued that mandatory use of DCTT could be ethical. If mandates increase adoption of DCTT and improve the public health response, this would reduce the likelihood of lockdowns, which are harmful and a severe limitation of individual liberty applied on a mass scale. On the other hand, mandated use of DCTT systems may not be effective. People may not adhere to the mandate by simply leaving their phone at home. Perhaps more important, should the technology not deliver the hoped-for benefits, having mandated the use of an unproven technology could result in a loss of public trust in the technology, in the entity instituting the mandate, and in the larger public health response, potentially leading to noncompliance with public health recommendations more broadly (Bernstein et al. 2019).

Any decision maker considering mandatory use, including government officials, institutional leaders, and employers, must convincingly address a number of considerations. Particularly important is the need to identify reliable evidence that the DCTT would be effective and to ensure that the burdens and benefits of use are equitable and justifiable. At this time, mandated use of DCTT by states or institutions is not justifiable given uncertainty about potential harms and benefits. Additional technology, user, and real-world testing is needed before mandatory use should be considered.

As with any public health effort, the amount of evidence that must be offered to illustrate that the intervention or program can achieve its aims, and the degree to which people should be able to exercise choice in their participation, should be in proportion to the anticipated burdens of the intervention or program. For example, the permissibility of mandating use of DCTT by the public depends on factors such as the sensitivity of the data that are collected, the extent to which public health is integrated within the DCTT system, and what actions are taken in response to confirmed virus exposure or being identified as COV+ (e.g., forced quarantine). The more burdens that are placed on individuals—for example, whether people are ordered into quarantine if they have been exposed to the virus, or if there are limited social supports for those in quarantine—the greater the demand should be on the performance of the DCTT system.

Perhaps the most effective way to generate widespread US adoption of DCTT will be to offer incentives for its use; in other contexts, generally speaking, small incentives have been shown to lead to an increase in desired outcome (Singer and Ye 2013; Lee et al. 2014). Given the importance of widespread use, modest incentives ought to be considered if and when there is sufficient evidence of the utility of DCTT, so long as those incentives are not mandates in disguise. Another "first line" approach to increasing use of DCTT is for trusted community leaders, public figures, health care professionals, and other respected individuals to communicate with the public and their communities about DCTT and to encourage its use through public engagement campaigns, if and when the technology demonstrates sufficient potential.

Establishing Meaningful Processes for
User Disclosure and Authorization (Consent)

Any effort to roll out DCTT should ensure that users have a meaningful opportunity to review and understand information about the specific technology and its uses. Moreover, given the importance of public trust and the current crisis of public trust in governments and technology companies handling private digital information, there is a strong ethics argument for requiring consent from individual users. We recommend a carefully crafted version of what is sometimes called simple consent, which consists of basic disclosure and voluntary agreement or authorization. This disclosure should include information about the purposes of the technology, the user's options for collecting and sharing data, purposes for which data can be used, and any known risks, among other information. This information should be presented in an accessible format on any DCTT app, and more detailed disclosures should be readily accessible for those who wish to review them.

Through an opt-in mechanism such as clicking a button to signal agreement, users should be able to indicate their intention to use a DCTT. The opt-in approach is consistent with mechanisms for agreement to use other downloaded applications. An opt-in approach should be part of the initial introduction of DCTT given the novelty of the technology and its uses and the need to build trust and confidence in the system. Successes of opt-out approaches in other areas suggest that the feasibility and value of an opt-out approach to DCTT should be carefully evaluated, particularly in conjunction with assessment of whether public health goals are being met (Rithalia et al. 2009). Such assessments should be informed by what is technologically possible, by local data regarding benefits and harms of the technology, and by evolving understanding of the degree to which an opt-out approach is likely to increase or decrease utilization among different populations.

Promoting Equity and Fairness in Application of DCTT

Digital contact tracing technology should be designed and used in ways that, as far as possible, promote an equitable distribution of benefits and burdens. DCTT should be deployed in a manner that does not propagate preexisting patterns of unfair disadvantage or distribute harms and risks unfairly throughout the population. It is well known that some communities have lower rates of technology and data access, and therefore may benefit less from use of DCTT unless steps are taken to address these digital disparities. Additionally, should use of DCTT be made a requirement for entry into a workplace, into a school, or onto transportation, then those who currently do not possess the required technology must not be unfairly burdened through lack of access. In order to mitigate this, states, localities, and institutions that recommend widespread use of DCTT should provide technology (e.g., mobile phones, Bluetooth devices) and free data packages to members of the community who desire but lack access to these devices.

Some populations may also experience greater harm, and greater fear of harm, from having their data collected. For example, some groups such as African Americans, Hispanic Americans, Muslim Americans, and undocumented immigrants have more reasonable fear of their data being handed over to law or immigration enforcement, and some groups have lower levels of trust in public health due to past injustices (Auxier et al. 2019; CSM 2017; Pew Research Center 2017; Rodrigues et al. 2018). This further substantiates the need to limit use of any data gathered by DCTT to its public health purpose.

Instituting Transparent Governance and Oversight

DCTT must be developed with an eye toward both present and future implications. We are rapidly gaining knowledge about SARS-CoV-2 and COVID-19, but still have essential gaps in our understanding. In the United States, public health responses including DCTT will generally be developed and coordinated by individual states, regional consortia (Reston, Sgueglia, and Mossburg 2020) and associations. Good governance in this context requires transparency and the creation of oversight bodies with the appropriate expertise and representation to allow nimble and effective responses while serving as trusted representatives.

In order to address the range of ethics and governance concerns that relate to the design and use of DCTT, we recommend that digital surveillance oversight committees be established, perhaps at a state level and with a platform for national coordination. These committees can provide ethics and regulatory review prior to and concurrent with widespread use of DCTT. The committees should be composed of a diverse group of experts capable of evaluating the quality of a DCTT system locally, including members of communities that experience higher rates of digital disparity.

When assessing the design and use of digital contact tracing systems, these committees (and the public more widely) should consider not only the risks and benefits accrued during the COVID-19 pandemic but also implications for the future. How can we navigate safe use of these technologies in a way that preserves public trust in them and enables the possibility of future beneficial use?

As a start, it should be emphasized that the principles offered in this and other guidance documents do not apply only during the pandemic. Future efforts to advance DCTT capabilities, during quieter times, should make every effort to follow them.

Introduction

Public health professionals around the world are working tirelessly to respond to the COVID-19 pandemic using tried-and-tested public health methods for infectious disease surveillance and control. These traditional methods are essential to the global COVID-19 response. To complement these actions and potentially augment the speed and efficacy of the public health workforce, digital technologies are being harnessed. Given the scale of the pandemic, significant efforts are being undertaken to develop and leverage public-facing and health-system-supportive technology solutions, including smartphone apps and other digital tools, that may aid public health surveillance and contact tracing.

Digital contact tracing technology and closely related digital health products (hereafter DCTT) have been used in several countries as part of broader disease surveillance and containment strategies. Globally, many digital COVID-19 contact tracing strategies have already emerged in response to the pandemic. This is not surprising given the ubiquity of mobile phones and other digital devices around the world ("Mobile Cellular Subscriptions (per 100 People)" 2018), experiences developed during prior outbreaks and pandemics, and the pre-COVID-19 momentum behind using digital technologies to support individual and health system capabilities (WHO 2017; Mathews et al. 2019; Aiello, Renson, and Zivich 2020; Mahmood et al. 2020). In the United States, DCTT has been proposed as an integral part of some plans to "reopen" the country (Allen et al. 2020; Hart et al. 2020; Simpson and Conner 2020). It is almost certain that these and related technologies will become part of not only the COVID-19 response but also the larger toolbox for future public health communicable disease prevention and control.

While novel public health surveillance technologies such as DCTT have theoretical promise, their effectiveness is unclear. These technologies also raise important ethical, legal, and governance challenges that require comprehensive analysis in order to support decision-making regarding their appropriate use. A number of frameworks, recommendations, and analyses have emerged recently in an effort to chart potentially "safe" pathways for use of public health disease surveillance technology. Many in the United States, such as the Electronic Frontier Foundation, Electronic Privacy Information Center, American Civil Liberties Union, and the Center for American Progress are proposing that digital public health surveillance technologies must embrace strict data privacy protections, decentralized data storage, a high degree of anonymity, and voluntary adoption (Crocker, Opsahl, and Cyphers 2020; Electronic Privacy Information Center 2020; Kahn Gilmor 2020; Simpson and Conner 2020). Others have argued that technologies that seek to enhance public health response during a pandemic should more closely align with the needs of public health professionals and the evidence-based procedures they follow, stating that interests in serving the public's health ought to weigh more heavily in the necessary balancing of stakeholder interests (de Jong et al. 2019; Watson et al. 2020). This view is in part based on a recognition that during countless other outbreaks, the public has benefited from traditional disease surveillance and contact tracing, which are heavily reliant on centralized data storage and, when necessary, the collection of identifiable information. These traditional approaches are governed by ethics principles (PHLS 2002), ethics guidelines (WHO 2017), and laws (ASTHO 2012), and digital technologies represent a new tool to support them.

While debates and recommendations about appropriate design and use of DCTT have focused intensely on minimizing important data-related risks, a wider lens is needed to fully appreciate the many additional critical questions that need attention. This report begins to grapple with these questions, which are critical to address in order to guide responsible use of DCTT. Given the complexity of the terrain, as a first step toward establishing a foundation for responsible decision-making regarding potential use of DCTT, we offer a set of guiding principles (see box). These principles are meant to apply to DCTT, as well as other digital technologies used in novel ways during pandemic response.

Guiding Principles for the Use of Digital
Public Health Technologies for Pandemic Response

Transparency and public engagement are essential to an inclusive digital public health response

- Government, public health, and digital technology leaders must engage effectively with the public and other stakeholders to communicate the utility, importance, oversight, and limitations of relevant digital technologies, including their implications for individuals' privacy and civil liberties.
- Transparency at all levels is essential for maintaining public trust and confidence.
- To the extent possible, digital public health responses should reflect the range of values that are important to individuals, including advancing the health and well-being of the community as a whole.
- Decision makers should recognize the sacrifices that some people may be willing to make during a pandemic in order to advance public health goals. Acceptance by some of particular monitoring capabilities should not be read as a willingness to extend these methods to other problems or uses.

Digital public health responses must represent the least infringement of civil liberties necessary to accomplish the public health goals

- If preferred digital public health strategies infringe on privacy and other civil liberties, the infringements must be sufficiently justified by the circumstances of the pandemic, offset by ample anticipated public benefit, and considered relative to infringements associated with other possible strategies, such as mass physical distancing.
- Only those data that are necessary and relevant for the stated public health purposes should be collected. Identifiable data should be stored in a secure manner and only for the period of time that the public health purposes require.
- Adopted technologies should not be used in ways that subject communities to discrimination or surveillance for non–public health reasons.
- Respect for individual autonomy requires that users are sufficiently informed of the public health goals of the technology and the extent to which those goals are being met.

Use of digital public health technologies and data must be guided by best available evidence

- Decisions to deploy digital public health technologies should be based on a careful assessment of the uses and limitations of any proposed technology, taking into account the best available evidence.

- Those who deploy digital public health technologies should continuously and systematically monitor their performance, as well as any evidence that is being generated in other contexts about the selected technological solution and about other competing technologies.
- Unintended consequences—including those that might impact public health goals, core values and interests of the public, and unfair advantage or disadvantage—should be carefully monitored and addressed as necessary.

Responsible use of digital public health technology requires meaningful governance and accountability

- Systems of governance must be trustworthy and well informed. They must be reviewed and adjusted as circumstances and evidence change or as unintended effects are identified.
- Trusted representatives who are capable of developing and implementing uniform and fair standards for adopting and utilizing underlying digital technology must be identified.
- Understandable, transparent, and publicly accessible rules must guide the collection, access, control, use, storage, and combination of data by government authorities, public and private institutions, and other parties such as public health researchers.
- Oversight, accountability, and consequences for abuse or misuse of these data must be explicit and enforceable.

The deployment of digital public health technology must be rooted in a commitment to equity

- Digital public health technologies should be deployed in a manner that does not propagate preexisting patterns of unfair disadvantage or further distribute harms and risks unfairly throughout the population.
- To the extent possible, digital public health technologies should be designed to rectify existing inequities.
- Oversight mechanisms must be in place to ensure that the improved public health outcomes are equitable and to detect and correct any unforeseen resultant injustices attributable to the technology or that can be addressed using the technology.
- The incentives and disincentives for adopting new technology must be equitable, not exploitative, and aligned with effective use of the technology.
- Disparity-driven technology gaps should be explicitly recognized. To the extent possible, provisions should be made to address the digital divide.

In reflecting on these principles, it becomes clear that if we wish not only to realize but to *maximize* the public good that might come from use of DCTT, we must carefully define and responsibly align public health needs and capabilities with technological needs and capabilities. We must understand that although technology may serve as a workforce multiplier, it alone will not solve the public health challenges we face. We must identify and address assumptions and misinformation about technologies and data use. We must provide the means and opportunity for informed decision-making by the public and those who serve as our representatives. Government officials, public health leaders, leaders of other institutions, employers, digital technology developers, and the public all must be adequately informed and engaged in order to make the best decisions possible under the circumstances.

ONE

Public Health Perspective

Types of Information Collected through Contact Tracing

Data Collected from Infected Persons

Symptoms and Course of Illness

Information about COVID-19 patients' signs, symptoms, and course of illness is important to public health because it provides a basis for refining clinical case definitions and informing health care providers and the general public (CDC 2020c). This includes the specific signs and symptoms manifested by persons who are COV+ as well as the relative frequency and durations of different signs and symptoms. This would also take into consideration those persons with no symptoms but who test positive—those who are presymptomatic (develop symptoms later), those who are postsymptomatic (clinically recovered but still infectious), and those who never manifest illness at all.

Typically, contact tracing begins with a case in which a person has confirmation of infection by means of a diagnostic test. However, in some cases test results are not reported until several days later and individuals may be identified as "presumptive positive" cases until testing can be completed. In these cases, contact tracing efforts will need to be updated when test results are returned. For example, if a test comes back negative, public health professionals will want to notify contacts that they no longer need to quarantine.

Movement and Contacts

In order to manage cases appropriately (identify and track the infected, isolate the sick, quarantine the exposed), public health officials need details on each case (Resolve to Save Lives, n.d.). First, they need to know who and where the individual is. That means personally identifiable information and contact information (address, phone numbers, email). It also means information about the nature, intensity, and duration of contact with individuals to whom they may have transmitted the disease. This may include information about where the individual works and the kind of work they do (e.g., health care worker), how they travel (e.g., bus, subway, car), and where they shop, or any other public venues they may have visited during a period of possible infectiousness (PIH 2020a). It may be helpful in certain circumstances for public health officials to ensure that suspected cases, contacts, or other high-risk individuals are following isolation and quarantine recommendations or orders.

Contact tracing involves identifying all individuals who have had significant exposure to confirmed or probable cases during the time prior to and after the onset of symptoms, both of which are times when the case is thought to be infectious (Africa CDC 2020). Contacts could be those who are caring for COVID-19 patients, especially if they lacked proper PPE, and those who had close interaction with the COV+ person over a sustained period of time, particularly in enclosed spaces (PIH 2020a). For COVID-19, contacts are identified by asking a person with a confirmed or probable case about people they may have been within 6 feet of for 15 minutes or more, starting from 48 hours before the onset of symptoms and lasting until the person is isolated (CDC 2020b).

Data Collected from Contacts of Infected Persons
Contact Details

In addition to the data collected from individuals with COVID-19, contact tracers will collect data from potentially exposed individuals (contacts). Information about the nature, intensity, and duration of contact with an infected person may be collected for a contact if information about the case is known to the contact. These details can help a contact tracer more accurately determine whether the contact is at high or low risk for SARS-CoV-2 transmission and help determine whether a contact should quarantine for 14 days (the upper bound of the SARS-CoV-2 incubation period). In addition, public health professionals may gather contacts' demographic information and other personal data to contribute to population-level disease surveillance and situational awareness about an epidemic (CDC 2005). However, the information needed at baseline is only a person's name and contact information.

Symptoms (If They Develop) and Course of Illness, as well as Information about Close Contacts

If a contact develops COVID-19 symptoms while in quarantine and/or tests positive for the virus, public health will then collect the data required for a COVID-19 case. This includes collecting information on the contacts that a person may have had (if any) in the days immediately before and during the course of their infection.

How Contact Tracing Information Informs Public Health Action

To reduce disease burden and help make "reopening" safer during the COVID-19 pandemic, the United States and other countries will need to identify, gather information about, and safely isolate cases and quarantine their contacts to reduce community transmission (Watson et al. 2020). Gathering information about possible cases and their contacts enables public health to break chains of transmission.

Contact tracing involves stages (CDC 2020a), including:

1. identifying an infected person as a COVID-19 case,

2. identifying the close contacts of that case (Africa CDC 2020),

3. getting in touch with contacts,

4. asking contacts to quarantine at home for 14 days,

5. assessing contacts for possible symptoms, and

6. following up with COV+ persons and their contacts to identify new or worsening symptoms and connect them with medical care if needed.

Contact tracers also play an important role in providing resources for COV+ persons who are in home isolation and their contacts who are in home quarantine. Knowing who and where cases and contacts are can enable provision of supplies, such as digital thermometers or masks. Effective contact tracing that enables isolated cases and quarantined contacts to remain at home also requires providing a range of social support services, or "care packages," from delivering food and medicines to trash pickup. Furthermore, vulnerable individuals who are homeless or otherwise unable to sufficiently isolate or quarantine in their current living conditions may need to have alternative housing arranged to safely remain separated from others (CDC 2020b).

Finally, contact tracers explain what quarantined contacts should do if they begin to develop symptoms consistent with COVID-19 (Africa CDC 2020). Depending on the context, contact tracers may engage in active monitoring by regularly communicating with contacts about their health status through phone, text message, or possibly mobile applications. In rare cases, public health can make quarantine mandatory and may monitor a quarantined individual to ensure that they do not break quarantine. Contact tracers may also facilitate access to health care by providing telemedicine resources or other information and support for accessing medical care.

Characteristics That Make Data Useful to Public Health for Reducing Disease Transmission

Data Access

If digital contact tracing technology and closely related digital health products (together DCTT) are intended to support the public health actions described above and directly amplify public health capacity to conduct case identification and contact tracing, then data collected through DCTT must be accessible to public health authorities. Identifying information and location data for cases and contacts of cases are necessary for public health use so that contact tracers can do their work to uncover ongoing transmission and enable isolation and quarantine. These data should also be durable, meaning that public health can return to the data in order to interact with and support cases and contacts. These data can also be useful at a population level, if de-identified and aggregated, by illuminating trends in community transmission and providing support for decisions about resource allocation.

Data Format

Data should be provided to public health authorities in a usable format that is compatible with public health systems and that has the granularity and specificity of personal information that is needed for use in contact tracing. Without personal identifiers, the data cannot be used by public health workers to undertake contact tracing. Data should also contain information about the nature of a contact, including the proximity of the contact and number of minutes that the person was in contact with an infected individual. Location data can also help public health authorities to conduct contact tracing, particularly when contact occurred in a crowded area and involved people who don't know one another. Location data from a case can help public health professionals identify contacts even when those contacts themselves are not using a contact tracing app because the data shows contact tracers where to look for additional contacts.

Data Accuracy

Data that identifies individuals as having sustained contact with a case must be as accurate as possible. If criteria for being considered a contact are too restrictive, it may result in missed contacts and sustained chains of disease transmission. If criteria are too broad, it may result in unnecessary restriction of movement, which could have significant personal and economic consequences.

Timeliness of Data

Data from cases and contacts must be timely in order to enable case-based management that will help reduce community transmission. For contact tracing to be effective, infected individuals need to be isolated, and their contacts identified and quarantined, as quickly as possible. Testing for SARS-CoV-2 can take time, sometimes many days for a test result. Especially because SARS-CoV-2 is transmissible during the pre-symptomatic period, data on symptomatic individuals should be made available to public health officials even before a positive test is returned in order to enable identification and quarantine of contacts right away. If this information is delayed until a test result is received, it may be too late to identify and quarantine contacts because contacts (if infected) will already be contagious and may have spread the virus to others.

The more that individuals opt to share their information to support contact tracing, the more effective contact tracing will be in breaking chains of viral transmission and controlling epidemics of COVID-19. The exact proportion of cases and contacts that need to be identified in order to avoid large surges of cases, which overwhelm health care systems, is uncertain, but the goal is to identify all infected cases and all close contacts of each case (PIH 2020b).

Recommendations

- Technologies or apps with the goal of enhancing public health capacity to identify cases and trace contacts in order to control the spread of SARS-CoV-2 should be designed to match functionality with that goal.

- Technologies or apps may produce some false negatives or false positives, but they should be accurate enough that public health authorities feel confident that they support, and don't detract from, contact tracing efforts.

- DCTT approaches for public health should be designed to facilitate the following:
  - identifying contacts, including those who may not be easily found otherwise;
  - finding and notifying contacts rapidly, before they develop symptoms if infected;
  - analyzing the nature of contact to determine whether contact is high, medium, or low risk, and to support decisions about whether a contact should quarantine; and
  - following up with cases and contacts so that public health can provide resources to support isolation and quarantine.

- Data collected through DCTT should be made available to public health professionals and to researchers in de-identified form to support population-level epidemiologic analysis.

TWO

Digital Technology and Contact Tracing

Characteristics of SARS-CoV-2
Relevant to Candidate Digital Solutions

The SARS-CoV-2 virus has some unique transmission characteristics and clinical manifestations that can help guide use of digital contact tracing solutions. Individuals infected with this virus may or may not show symptoms, or may show a range of different and sometimes nonspecific symptoms. Estimates regarding the percentage of individuals who are infected but never develop symptoms is highly uncertain, ranging from 5% to 50% (Heneghan, Brassey, and Jefferson 2020). Data suggest that a substantial proportion of transmissions—perhaps as high as 50%—occur between individuals who are not symptomatic and that transmissibility may extend out as long as 3 days before the onset of symptoms (WHO 2020).

The complexity of asymptomatic and presymptomatic transmission makes it more difficult to identify all cases of COVID-19. It also means that manual contact tracing is less effective because people are unlikely to remember all of their contacts during the long period of infectivity (Ferretti et al. 2020); however, it does not negate the need for contact tracing. Identifying symptomatic cases will still help greatly with slowing the spread because their contacts can be asked to quarantine to prevent them from spreading the virus if they are indeed infected. This means that whether they become symptomatic or not, contacts will be quarantined and the chain of transmission will be broken. If contact tracing can be implemented on a large enough scale, perhaps with support from DCTT, eventually the virus could be managed at much lower levels of community transmission, and large epidemics of unrecognized spread will not occur.

The transmissibility of the virus when a person has no symptoms further suggests that effective solutions may require multimodal interventions, combining contact tracing with frequent, rapid, and ubiquitous testing and continued social distancing to varying extents (Cheng et al. 2020).

Because of presymptomatic spread, contact tracing efforts and digital solutions to augment those efforts should support identification of contacts a person had 2 days before their symptoms and at least 3 days after the resolution of those symptoms (if the person continued to have contacts through that time period) (CDC 2020d). Additionally, public health messages delivered by these technologies should urge contacts to quarantine for the full 14-day incubation period.

Previously Existing Contact Tracing Technologies

Prior to this pandemic, health agencies in high-, medium-, and low-income countries had begun to develop and use digital tools to augment the management of infectious diseases including sexually transmitted infections (HIV, chlamydia, gonorrhea) and high-consequence epidemics (Ebola) (Danquah et al. 2019)). However, these have been primarily used to facilitate case interviews, partner notification (in the case of STIs), and record keeping, as opposed to fully digitizing or automating the contact tracing process.

It has been recently suggested that digital contact tracing could contribute to the management of the ongoing COVID-19 pandemic, and the experiences of containing SARS-CoV-2 in countries such as China, Singapore, and South Korea provide noteworthy examples. However, undertaking this case-based intervention on the scale required to achieve pandemic control is a novelty in the history of public health. Although technological development is proceeding rapidly, several foundational issues have yet to be resolved, including functionality, connectivity to public health authorities and informatics systems, usability by disease intervention specialists (DIS, also referred to as contact tracers), and sufficient protection of personally identifiable information, among others.

Digital contact tracing technologies and platforms have recently been introduced, and the CDC has published preliminary criteria for evaluating these tools (CDC 2020e). It can be helpful to consider three broad approaches along the spectrum of potential methods of digital contact tracing: a maximal approach (typified by the South Korean government's centralized data collection (M. S. Kim 2020)); a minimal approach (typified by the Apple/Google decentralized privacy-protecting proximity tracking (Apple and Google n.d.)); and a diverse middle ground that aims to augment manual contact tracing with the collection of digital data. Perhaps the most promising approach in this middle ground involves allowing users to turn over both proximity data and GPS location data (i.e., cell-site location data) to public health authorities on a voluntary basis.

Along with this "minimal to maximal" spectrum in the design of digital contact tracing technologies and systems, there is another spectrum that concerns voluntary versus mandatory use of these technologies: are individuals entirely free to use these technologies or not, or should policies incentivize or even mandate their use? At one extreme, South Korea (Republic of Korea) implemented a system (called Safe Korea) supported by the Ministry of the Interior and Safety that collects a variety of personal data in a centralized database in order to enforce quarantine orders and track possible contacts (M. S. Kim 2020). Israel also implemented a centralized involuntary data collection system for tracking COVID-19 cases and alerting those who may have been exposed (Hendrix and Eglash 2020). In Poland, health authorities have set up mandatory "check-ins" involving a GPS-waypoint capture and "selfie" photographs sent to the monitoring agency to ensure that individuals are not breaking quarantine (Hamilton 2020).

These centralized systems can be designed to incorporate data from a variety of sources. The data collected include location data from mobile phones. QR codes can also be scanned to track the use of public transit where GPS data may be inadequate (due to low resolution) to accurately distinguish the occupants of one vehicle from another. The data collected from mobile phones can then be integrated with data from other sources, such as facial-recognition cameras, credit card transactions, and social media.

At the other extreme of technology invasiveness for contact tracing, isolation, and quarantine, many corporations and working groups (including the Apple/Google collaboration) have developed privacy-preserving proximity tracking (PPPT) using Bluetooth Low Energy (BLE) "handshakes" that record close contact between mobile phone users. In most architectures, these proximity data are stored in the users' phones as anonymized "beacons" that cannot be used to re-identify the users directly. If a user with a PPPT app installed on their phone tests positive and enters test results into their app, those who have been identified as having been in close proximity to them can be notified by the app. This notification can be automatic or at the discretion of the person who is COV+, depending on the app design. If notified, a user who has been in contact with a COV+ individual would receive a push notification alerting them to possible exposure (which may be timestamped), but with no other identifying information.

Because of its reliance on anonymized data, PPPT on its own is distinct from manual contact tracing. In recognition of this fact, some designers and researchers now use the more descriptive term "exposure notification." Moreover, the public health usefulness of PPPT is uncertain: it is unclear how PPPT can best be used in tandem with manual contact tracing, especially if the data it collects are inaccessible to or unusable by public health authorities. It remains to be seen whether PPPT will provide significant benefit operating alongside but not integrated into manual contact tracing.

Between these extremes, there are a number of possible middle-ground approaches that aim to strike a balance among public health utility, technological feasibility, and user privacy protections. This middle ground divides into two rough categories: centralized storage of de-identified data and decentralized storage of personally identifying data. The United Kingdom's NHSX is reportedly developing an app that would utilize BLE handshakes to collect anonymized proximity data, which would then be stored on a centralized, government-operated server.

The most prevalent middle-ground approach in the United States context involves the collection and storage of personal data—including identifying information and location data—on the user's phone. This decentralized but personally identifiable data can then be voluntarily shared with public health officials if the user tests positive for SARS-CoV-2. For example, an MIT team has developed an app called Private Kit: Safe Paths (MIT n.d.) that stores users' location data on their phone for 28 days. If a user tests positive, she can voluntarily upload her location data to a website that is accessible only to public health officials. Officials can then analyze this personally identifiable data and, subsequently, broadcast redacted and de-identified data to other users. Healthy users would have access to these redacted location data of COV+ users, but their own data would not leave their phones. (The developers plan to incorporate BLE proximity data once available.) Along similar lines, the North Dakota state government has rolled out an app that stores both location data and proximity data on a user's phone, which can be voluntarily released by the user to public health authorities if the user tests positive (NDDoH 2020). At a minimum, the storage of user location data can function as a "memory aid" if the user tests positive. But releasing the data to public health authorities may help them analyze the spread of COVID-19 and alert individuals or groups that have been in contact with persons who are COV+. An overview of various DCTT apps and platforms, as well as features that are relevant to this analysis, are provided in Table 1.

Because DCTTs are so new, very little is known about their actual utility to public health authorities for controlling this pandemic. Although multiple countries that have had success in greatly reducing transmission of SARS-CoV-2 have included DCTT in their response, these countries have employed multiple simultaneous approaches to controlling the virus, including manual contact tracing, and it is difficult to disentangle what made those responses successful. Preliminary impressions from Iceland may suggest that DCTT, at least in that context, had a small impact on reducing transmission, "especially compared with methods of manual contact tracing, such as phone calls" (Hadavas 2020). This is with the highest public download rate of any DCTT app thus far.

DCTTs have the potential to be helpful, but they also have the potential to distract from other public health efforts, including manual contact tracing. Concerns about implementation of DCTT from the public health perspective include that data generated may not be useful to public health authorities, either because they don't include detailed data to aid contact tracers or because the data are inaccurate (Mills Rodrigo 2020). DCTT, if not calibrated well, could be overly inclusive and create many false positives. This would be harmful to those individuals being notified and

TABLE 1 Examples of Digital Contact Tracing Technologies to Support Active Public Health Surveillance, and Relevant Features

Intervention Type	App Name	Developer or Country	Purpose: Proximity-based exposure notification	Purpose: Digital contact tracing (DCT)	Tech: Bluetooth LE	Tech: GPS	Tech: SMS	Data Storage: Centralized	Data Storage: Decentralized	Participation: Mandatory (actually or functionally)	Participation: Voluntary/opt-in	Government access
Max	WeChat / Alipay	China	✓		✓	✓		✓		✓		Data comes from government sources; location data sent to police
Middle Ground	Trace Together	Singapore		✓	✓				✓		✓	Mandatory government access if positive
Middle Ground	NHSX/Oxford	Oxford		✓	✓			✓			✓	Government maintains data
Middle Ground	NextTrace	Fred Hutchinson Cancer Research Center		✓			✓				✓	Government maintains data, but no storage
Middle Ground	COVID SafePaths	MIT		✓	✓	✓			✓		✓	Voluntary upload by users who test positive
Middle Ground	Aarogya Setu	India		✓	✓	✓		✓	✓		✓	Anonymized, aggregate
Middle Ground	Care19	North Dakota		✓	✓	✓		✓	✓		✓	In aggregate; optional if positive
Minimal	CovidSafe	Univ of Washington	✓	✓	✓				✓		✓	None
Minimal	CovidWatch	Univ of Stanford & Univ of Waterloo		✓	✓				✓		✓	To validate test results
Minimal	CoEpi	CoEpi	✓		✓	✓			✓		✓	Opt-in to share BT and symptom log with CoEpi server
Minimal	ito	Germany	✓		✓				✓		✓	None; positive results to ito server

asked to quarantine unnecessarily, and it could result in large proportions of the population remaining at home at any one time. Individuals living or working in congregate settings could receive frequent notifications that would result in their inability to leave quarantine for long periods of time. Finally, public health authorities could also become inundated by data from these technologies and not have sufficient approaches to manage or analyze the incoming information.

Relevant Differences between Manual and Digital Contact Tracing

There are several noteworthy differences between manual contact tracing efforts and use of DCTT. First, there is a significant amount of evidence regarding the effectiveness of manual contact tracing, which is lacking for DCTT. Second, manual contact tracers interact with individuals who are confirmed or suspected cases and contacts of cases, but not other members of the general public; DCTT intervention would affect all users regardless of circumstances (though some more than others). Third, manual contact tracing occurs most often through human-to-human encounters, with the opportunity to clarify misconceptions, address worries, and express sympathy and other important affects; DCTT can certainly incorporate sharing of important information and potentially communicate some affect, but it currently lacks a range of other human capabilities and characteristics. Fourth, there typically are fewer data intermediaries in manual contact tracing (fewer entities handling data); in DCTT, a valid argument could be made that a wide range of technology developers (and perhaps mobile network operators) must remain connected to relevant data in order to continuously identify problems and improve functionality.

It is because of these and other differences that DCTT has been proposed as a potential complement to, rather than a replacement for, manual contact tracing. However, over time it is possible that technology could develop to close gaps between some of these differences (if and as needed), and, in parallel, the goals of contact tracing and public health surveillance may evolve.

THREE

Ethics of Designing and Using DCTT

Those developing DCTT, and those considering its use, should systematically take into account and document alignment with the guiding principles outlined in this report.

When considering the ethics of DCTT, key ethical questions concern the features that DCTT should have (e.g., should digital contact tracing apps collect users' location data?), whether and how individuals' data should be shared with public health authorities, how ethically to encourage use of DCTT (e.g., under what circumstances would it be ethical to incentivize or mandate use of DCTT), what kind of supports and equity-promoting measures should accompany use of DCTT, and how governance and oversight of DCTT should be structured.

The sections that follow consider these questions one by one. A key conclusion of this report is that these features of the design and use of DCTT are ethically interrelated—reaching a determination regarding any one question requires careful consideration of them all. Rather than reaching "one size fits all" conclusions about specific features of uses of DCTT, decision makers should ethically assess DCTT systems holistically.

Generally, a public health measure is ethically justifiable if it strikes a reasonable balance between competing considerations and if it provides sufficient public health benefit (or the prospect of benefit) to justify the burdens associated with it. DCTT systems are ethically justifiable if they strike a reasonable balance between multiple ethical considerations including:

- enabling an effective and efficient public health response,
- protecting individual privacy and preventing harms to individuals,

including harms from sensitive data being revealed and from erroneously being subjected to isolation or quarantine orders,

- allowing individuals to control what information about them is collected and revealed to whom, including through appropriate disclosure and authorization processes for data collection,

- promoting equitable distribution of benefits and burdens of DCTT,

- maintaining public trust in DCTT and in the COVID-19 public health response, and

- taking seriously the future implications of decisions that we make today.

To illustrate a holistic assessment, consider whether it is ethically justifiable for an employer to mandate that employees use a DCTT as a condition of returning to work. This will depend upon many features of the DCTT system: what kind of data the DCTT collects (e.g., does it collect location data or just record proximity events); whether there is public health capacity to make good use of these data; what the data are used for (e.g., will the employer ban an employee from the workplace on the basis of a DCTT-identified contact?); what kind of social supports are available (e.g., is there paid leave for employees?); what employees' attitudes are toward use of DCTT; and whether mandating use is likely to have public health benefit, among other factors. These factors may vary from place to place and may change over the course of the pandemic. Thus there is no "one size fits all" ethically optimal approach to DCTT.

Justifying the Use of DCTT Systems

A foundational issue is why deploying *any* DCTT during a pandemic is justified, given there are manual contact tracing capabilities that are well established, while the performance and effectiveness of novel technologies is less established. The need to move quickly to minimize the spread of the virus poses challenges here, as the data needed to fully make the case that these technologies substantially contribute to the public health response may not be available prior to widespread use. The primary argument for DCTT is that the capacity of manual contact tracing may be exceeded, and we may not be able to bolster the public health workforce rapidly and sufficiently enough to meet needs. DCTT has the potential to quickly and exponentially expand the reach of contact tracing. In addition, DCTT may allow more efficient identification and quarantine of potential contacts of COV+ people than manual contact tracing alone, particularly given the high number of infections that have been spread by asymptomatic individuals.

Nonetheless, reasonable people disagree about the prudence of pursuing DCTT, especially given its limited performance history and potential risks, including diverting attention and resources from more effective interventions. The limited attention and resources available during a pandemic must be allocated efficiently and effectively.

To justify potentially widespread use of technologies such as DCTT, therefore, a number of considerations must be addressed:

- whether the technology is designed to meet an important and unmet public health need,
- whether there is sufficient evidence or reason to suggest that the technology will be effective at serving its purpose,
- whether the outbreak is characterized by sufficiently severe morbidity and mortality and a high rate of disease transmission to warrant large-scale introduction of novel systems,
- whether there are other less autonomy-restricting or less risky alternatives to widespread use, and
- whether it is reasonably likely that a sufficient number of individuals will use the technology to achieve the intended public health benefit.

Monitoring and Evaluating Technologies to Inform Policy and Practice

A number of public health ethics principles necessitate the ongoing monitoring and evaluation of DCTT systems. First, DCTT must be shown to perform reasonably well at achieving its stated goal: reducing the spread of SARS-CoV-2. The effectiveness of DCTT programs should be illustrated at a number of stages.

1. Robust initial technology testing is needed to publicly justify the widespread adoption of DCTT and avoid public failures, which may hamper future uptake (e.g., Lovejoy 2020; Morse 2020). This typically includes alpha testing in virtual environments and beta testing in different community settings.

2. If and when a DCTT is implemented on a wide scale, it must be monitored on an ongoing basis to assess reach, effectiveness, functionality, best practices, and any harms.

3. When approaching a previously identified stopping point for use of DCTT, monitoring can help to identify when utilization is no longer needed.

If at any of these points evidence clearly suggests harm (particularly in comparison to other methods that the public might find more acceptable), this evidence should provide a basis upon which to revisit strategies, priorities, and allocation of resources. Attention should be given to foreseeable side effects that may dramatically influence the overall effectiveness of the program, such as individuals carrying their smartphones around with them selectively so as to avoid particular undesired consequences of DCTT policies.

Anonymized aggregate data, including user feedback, must be evaluated to ensure that benefits and burdens are distributed fairly. As noted earlier, unintended burdens may include inequitable outcomes that may arise in a DCTT program; for example, resulting from uneven access to the required technology to participate, disparate concerns about surveillance within some communities that might limit widespread use, or discrimination that may result from being identified as COV+ due to the program or for communities that are termed "hotspots" based on maps of COV+ location data. Additionally, it is possible that some communities might get higher rates of false positives because they are located in densely populated areas, thus increasing the burden of self-isolation. If any of these inequities are identified, steps must be taken to mitigate them.

Finally, numerous actors should engage in the monitoring and evaluation of DCTT systems. Technology developers and public health researchers have a clear role in this process. Technology developers should work with public health researchers to monitor accuracy, precision, functionality, confidence of estimates, sources of error, and the like. Researchers may also be able to contribute innovative methods to systematically and rapidly evaluate candidate technologies, such as by deploying cluster randomized stepped wedge (Hemming et al. 2015) or adaptive trial designs and techniques (e.g., response-adjusted randomization) (Pallmann et al. 2018). These approaches were also proposed for use in research to assign candidate experimental treatments and vaccines during the 2014-15 Ebola outbreak (Berry et al. 2016). When formal research activities are pursued, ethics principles and legal requirements for the conduct of research should apply (e.g., The Belmont Report).

Furthermore, any workplace or institution that incentivizes or mandates use of DCTT has a responsibility to provide evidence that the intervention, at minimum, is not likely to cause harm and to monitor for unanticipated burdens. In all cases, it is vital that a trusted intermediary be involved in the evaluation of DCTT programs to limit perceptions of bias and ensure a legitimate basis for decision-making. Nonsensitive aggregate DCTT analyses should be made available to the public so as to permit verification and inform continuing public debates about its usefulness and necessity. At an individual level, data should be available to users that would permit them to further investigate their personal risk with public health officials or other health workers. This is important not only to ensure their health and well-being but also to add a layer of protection against unnecessary quarantine.

Recommendations

- Reviews of DCTT systems must be conducted in part by an independent intermediary that has established the public's trust.

- Those who authorize use of DCTT within a particular jurisdiction or institution should continuously and systematically monitor the technology's performance in that context. This should include monitoring for effectiveness and benefit, monitoring for harms, and monitoring for the fair distribution of both benefits and harms. They should also monitor evidence that is being generated in other contexts about their selected technological solution and about other competing technologies.

- Data should be available to users that would permit them to further investigate their personal risk with public health officials or other health workers to add a layer of protection against unnecessary quarantine.

Public Trust and Public Attitudes

Researchers have estimated, perhaps conservatively, that DCTT use by 80% of smartphone owners—56% of the population—will be needed to suppress the epidemic (Hinch et al. 2020). These estimates also highlight that some decrease in transmission would be realizable even with lower rates of technology adoption. As such, in order to maximize impact, it is essential to gain a thorough understanding of public perspectives on DCTT, including which features and uses of the technology the public finds acceptable, which kinds of DCTT the public would be most likely to use, and which designs and uses of DCTT would maintain or jeopardize public confidence and trust. There will be variation in public attitudes within and across societies and over time.

With respect to what we currently know about public attitudes and trust in DCTT in the United States, polling data suggest some potential support and also some divisions regarding willingness to use the technology. Polls conducted by groups based at the University of Zurich (Hargittai et al. 2020) and the University of Oxford (Altmann et al. 2020) suggest that more than 60% of Americans would be willing to install such an app. Both a Washington Post–University of Maryland poll (2020) and a Kaiser Family Foundation poll (Kirzinger et al. 2020) show roughly half of the population would be willing to install the app. Over half of the population (59%) would be willing to share their COVID-19 positive test result with an app in order to anonymously share that information with their contacts (Washington Post–UMD 2020). Only 29% of respondents to a March 12–27 Oliver Wyman Forum poll (Elliott et al. 2020) said that they would be willing to share their location data. Additionally, Washington Post–UMD data and Pew data from 2019 suggest that approximately one in six Americans do not have a smartphone and thus cannot use the technology without intervention (Pew Research Center 2020).

People may be more willing, however, to download an app if it will ease social distancing policies and allow for more economic and social activity. Willingness to install a contact tracing app increased among respondents to the Kaiser Family Foundation poll from 50% to 66% when respondents were asked if they would be willing to do so to allow schools and businesses to reopen. Additionally, who develops or administers the app appears to matter. Respondents to the Washington Post–UMD poll indicated higher levels of trust that their anonymity would be preserved by public health agencies and universities than by tech companies or health insurance companies. Further, more respondents to the Oliver Wyman Forum poll were willing to share their health information with public health authorities (55%) than the local government (35%), their employer or school (33%), or the federal government (27%).

These data suggest that people will be more willing to use a contact tracing app when the potential benefits are clearly identified and valued, such as lifting social distancing measures, and they will be more willing to do so if the data are going to a public health agency rather than the federal government or a tech company. Other factors that seem to be associated with greater willingness to install a contact tracing app include younger age and the app source (Hargittai et al. 2020), with a preference for apps distributed by public health agencies over others such as health insurers or public universities (Hargittai and Redmiles 2020). However, all of this must be read with caution, as public polling may not be representative of some populations or of widespread public attitudes. Further, these attitudes may shift over time and may be discordant with behaviors (Barth and de Jong 2017).

Deliberative public engagement efforts would be an appropriate means of filling in gaps in understanding about the acceptability of different approaches (Fishkin and Laslett 2003; Cavalier 2011). In addition, including the public, particularly in the earlier stages of planning a path to sustainable resolution to the pandemic, could serve to help disseminate a nuanced understanding of what is at stake, including the key challenges and trade-offs. Aggregated public polling results are not sufficient as a proxy for careful analyses of the ethical challenges; but, they do provide a necessary input for these analyses. Integrating lessons and outputs from public engagement into guidance and other products requires special attention and should be validated and enhanced through further engagement.

- More research into public attitudes is needed. In particular, in-depth qualitative research should examine public attitudes about perceptions of trust in DCTT among different communities, which features of DCTT influence trust, and the extent to which people are willing to provide different types of data through DCTT to help their community.

- States and localities that are considering adopting DCTT should engage with the public to increase their understanding of the acceptability of DCTT design features and uses among diverse communities.

Designing Flexible Technology to Maximize Public Health Utility While Respecting Other Values

Values in Design

Efforts to advance DCTT in the United States and elsewhere have emphasized the importance of "privacy by design"; that is, building privacy and security protections into the design of technology, rather than counting on responsible use alone (Cavoukian 2010). As noted above, some major technology companies have signaled this position through development of decentralized privacy-preserving proximity tracking (PPPT) systems. These systems embed features such as decentralization, anonymity of users, bans on collection of location data, and minimal reliance on or integration of public health authorities or other government actors. Many of these features have also been embraced early by advocacy organizations (Crocker, Opsahl, and Cyphers 2020; Electronic Privacy Information Center 2020; Kahn Gilmor 2020) and in an open letter from nearly 300 researchers ("Joint Statement on Contact Tracing" 2020).

Privacy by design provides principles that incorporate one set of values (privacy) into the design of DCTT. Importantly, the principles acknowledge the need to design privacy defaults into systems, while maintaining the capacity of those systems to achieve their otherwise justifiable ends. Put another way, privacy by design "embraces legitimate non-privacy objectives and accommodates them, in an innovative positive-sum manner" (Cavoukian 2010, p. 4).

This stance, simple in its statement, is not easy to satisfy. Given that "objectives" are themselves driven by values, it begs for an articulation of additional values (aside from privacy) that individuals and groups within society—including many privacy advocates—may believe to be important. For example, at any moment, in addition to valuing their own privacy, individuals may value efficiency, equity, autonomy, economic well-being, companionship, patriotism, or solidarity. Moreover, the above stance necessitates an acknowledgment that peoples' value priorities often change when circumstances change, not least of which during a pandemic when mass physical distancing has made it difficult to fully realize many important values (aside from physical privacy). A different orientation is needed at this moment. As Flanagan, Howe, and Nissenbaum (2008) conceptualized in 2008, we should take a "values in design" approach to DCTT—an approach that designs a broader range of values, such as those enumerated above, into technology.

This approach requires a wider ethical lens through which to examine DCTT and requires hard but important work to appropriately balance competing interests within technology architecture. For example, there is value in technology providing users the option to collect their location history and share it with public health professionals in order to advance the public health response, increase system efficiencies (e.g., by contributing information that can lead to better data processing), and reduce the burden on essential workers. For some, this might be an expression of autonomy, solidarity, or patriotism. At the same time, there is value in further advancing autonomy by designing technology to allow individuals to control what data about them are collected and shared.

Justifying a Middle-Ground Approach to DCTT

We ought to embrace a DCTT that has a default of interoperability and privacy protection, but that does not stop there. Triggering events, such as entry of a positive test result or receipt of a notification that one was proximate to someone who tested positive, could, for example, generate a push notification that users can acknowledge in order to permit transmission of potentially useful location data to public health authorities. This could be accompanied by an explanation of the value of the information and relevant restrictions on its use.

At this point, it is worth reiterating that manual contact tracing—

which involves collecting information from people who've tested positive and their contacts—includes collection of personal information and potentially embarrassing or sensitive data about the places they've been and the people they've had contact with. Manual contact tracing efforts use these data to uncover ongoing transmission, provide useful information tailored to the individual, and enable isolation and quarantine as necessary.

It stands to reason that if these forms of data can be collected by a DCTT and provided to public health authorities in a maximally secure and voluntary way (with clear rules regarding authorized uses), this may amplify public health authorities' manual contact tracing efforts. For example, location data from DCTT could help jog people's memories about where they've been and fill in memory gaps. This is especially relevant given the long period of infectivity of SARS-CoV-2, which begins before people are symptomatic and therefore before they are aware they are infected (Ferretti et al. 2020). Location data might reveal that a COV+ person was at a restaurant at an exact time and date, which could be followed up by contact tracers, who could alert the public or use other measures to reach those who were also present in the restaurant at the same time. In other disease contexts (see Furlanello et al. 2002; Dredze et al. 2013; Eckhoff and Tatem 2015; Fraccaro et al. 2019), geolocation data have demonstrated some potential to support epidemiology and disease surveillance, with technical cautions regarding accuracy and the like (Beukenhorst et al. 2017).

These benefits are currently speculative for DCTT. At present, providing public health authorities with large amounts of data on cases and potential case contacts will be useful only if there is sufficient public health capacity to follow up on these data. In addition, there is a risk of low-quality data from DCTT flooding the system. Investigating potential case contacts identified by a DCTT may distract them from other important efforts and at some point overwhelm public health capacity altogether. Whether and to what extent data from DCTT will benefit contact tracing efforts is unknown, pointing again to the importance of continuously collecting high-quality evidence about DCTT.

Nevertheless, what would enable the most flexible and potentially robust public health response is to design DCTT so that restricted data sharing is possible. From an ethics perspective, the collection and use of sensitive data in manual contact tracing efforts (described above) is typically seen as ethically justifiable so long as there is sufficient public health benefit and need. Thus, wouldn't it seem appropriate from both a public health and ethics perspective to design DCTT systems to enable similar data to be shared with public health authorities when and if there is ethical justification for sharing them?

Why, instead, do so many advocate that DCTT should be designed as a "minimal" system, when this arguably ties the hands of public health and individual users and precludes the collection of data that public health authorities (and indeed many other apps on our phones) typically collect? We here consider, and appraise, some of the reasons that may motivate individuals and groups to argue for minimalistic positions:

1. **Proponents of minimal systems may believe that such systems will be most widely adopted.** Some groups have maintained that only these systems will earn and maintain public trust and be widely adopted (Simpson and Conner 2020). For example, the previously referenced open letter ("Joint Statement on Contact Tracing" 2020) asserts: "Some of the Bluetooth-based proposals respect the individual's right to privacy, whilst others would enable (via mission creep) a form of government or private sector surveillance that would catastrophically hamper trust in and acceptance of such an application by society at large. It is crucial that citizens trust the applications in order to produce sufficient uptake to make a difference in tackling the crisis. It is vital that, in coming out of the current crisis, we do not create a tool that enables large scale data collection on the population, either now or at a later time. Thus, solutions which allow reconstructing invasive information about the population should be rejected without further discussion."

   Response: While it is true that public trust in and acceptance of DCTT is essential for its success, there is insufficient evidence that public trust would be threatened by a DCTT system that has the capacity to collect location data and enable voluntary sharing of those data with public health authorities. A contrasting perspective is that maintaining public trust requires maintaining public confidence that the DCTT system is providing useful information, is benefiting and not harming individuals, and is advancing the public health response (Leprince-Ringuet 2020). From this perspective, a system that is less well integrated into the broader public health response, or that generates a higher rate of false positives (as some suggest decentralized approaches might (Fraser et al. 2020)), may fare worse when it comes to maintaining public confidence and trust.

2. **Proponents may hold the view that minimal systems are harmless (or nearly harmless) to individuals.** This is because individuals are anonymous, none of their location data are gathered, and none of their identifiable data are shared with anyone. In contrast, DCTT systems that collect and share identifiable data, including location data, may be seen as posing risks of harm to individuals.

> **Response:** While minimal systems may be harmless (or nearly harmless) from the perspective of protecting privacy, they may not be harmless from the perspective of public health if they generate system inefficiencies through producing too many false positive or false negative contacts. Aside from presenting a challenge for public health professionals, false positives could also harm individuals. If users receive a large volume of automated messages alerting them to proximity events, will this cause distress? Will a large volume of alerts cause users to become disengaged and stop using the DCTT or lose confidence in contact tracing more generally as a legitimate method of disease control? Admittedly, these are just potential harms and risks; it is unknown the degree to which they will materialize. The point is that privacy-related harms are not the only relevant harms to individuals that we should consider when assessing DCTT.
>
> We acknowledge the risk under a middle-ground DCTT of data being used in ethically unjustifiable and harmful ways. For example, it would be against the principles and recommendations articulated in this report for data to be sold or monetized by technology companies or others for corporate gain, and this misuse of data would be more intrusive if the data were potentially identifiable. What makes it ethically justifiable to take this risk is the compensating benefit of allowing the most flexible and robust public health

response during the pandemic, but this alone is not sufficient. The risk of inappropriate uses must be reduced by ensuring stringent requirements for data security and access, as well as clear legal protections and recourse for any violations (as discussed further below).

3. **Proponents may believe that DCTT systems should not collect location data as this would be too intrusive and of insufficient value.** Some proponents of PPPT systems maintain that recording proximity events is sufficient, and data relating to users' movement and location should not be collected (Ingram 2020). The thought may be: all we need to know is whether two individuals came into close enough contact for viral transmission to have occurred; we don't need to know where or when this contact occurred, and there is no need to collect and store users' location data.

   Response: This conclusion might be too hasty. As discussed above, there is potential (though unproven) benefit to providing public health authorities with location data. Location data could help jog people's memories about where they've been, provide more context for understanding the nature of "proximity events" captured by the DCTT, and allow public health authorities to quickly define a category of individuals who may be at risk. Collecting location data from cases is what public health authorities do on a regular basis, following best practices for manual contact tracing.

   In addition, many people's location data are currently gathered by apps on their phones and used for various purposes, such as to provide more accurate navigation, to offer entertainment, or to improve services. Many are willing to accept these capabilities because they provide some value in return. Why not allow DCTT to also collect these data so that the data are available for users to share with public health officials, who can then do their work more effectively and refine their understanding of how the disease transmits? If many are willing to have these data used to find a better route home, why not let individuals share these data to support the effort to save lives?

4. **Proponents may hold the view that minimal systems pose little or no threat to individual autonomy, whereas systems that collect identifiable data and integrate public health do pose a threat to individual autonomy.** For example, they may worry that use of DCTT could be mandated and not a voluntary choice, and in this circumstance mandatory use of minimal DCTT would be less intrusive, risky, and privacy violating. Another worry might be that it's theoretically possible that DCTT could share individuals' data with public health authorities without users' full understanding; if the technology does not even gather identifiable data, then it's not possible for these data to be shared without the individual's consent.

> **Response:** We discuss the importance of appropriately designed disclosures and consent below, as well as the high bar that would need to be met to ethically justify mandatory use. At this time, mandated use of DCTT by states or institutions is not justifiable, given uncertainty about potential harms and benefits. Users should have a meaningful opportunity to review and understand information about the specific technology and its uses and to consent. Assuming that individuals are not required to use DCTT and that they provide consent to using it, designing DCTT to make data collection and sharing possible is the design choice that maximizes individual autonomy, because it provides individuals with options they may value.
>
> Individuals may wish to share their data with public health authorities for both self-interested and altruistic reasons. For example, someone who has tested positive for SARS-CoV-2 and enters this test result into an app may wish to be connected to public health authorities in order to be provided with needed information, resources, and support. She may wish for public health authorities to be provided with her phone number in case they need to reach her to provide additional information. Further, someone who has been alerted by an app that he had a "proximity event" with a person who has tested positive for SARS-CoV-2 may wish he had location data to share with public health authorities in order to help ascertain whether this event is a cause for concern or whether it is likely a false positive (e.g., he and the COV+ person were sepa-

rated by a wall). Someone who tests positive for the virus may also wish to share their location history with public health authorities in order to be as helpful as possible to the overall public health response by facilitating de-identified aggregate analyses that identify locations of higher transmission or contribute to refining overall understanding of the disease and pandemic.

5. **Concerns about "surveillance creep" and the long-term downstream effects of digital contact tracing system may also motivate embrace of minimal DCTT.** Digital contact tracing technology that collects identifiers and location data and has the capacity to share them with public health authorities may represent a massive and concerning increase in government surveillance of the public. It might be feared that the use of this surveillance capacity in the COVID-19 response sets an unwelcome precedent for future use in other contexts. Designing DCTT as minimal systems may be a way to minimize the risk of surveillance creep and to minimize the harms associated with potential future uses of the technology.

> **Response:** Surveillance creep is a serious concern. To guard against surveillance creep, protections should be put in place to ensure that only those data that are necessary and relevant for the public health purposes at hand are collected and used, and data should be kept only for the period of time needed for those public health purposes. In the face of these concerns, it is important to emphasize that widespread use of DCTT in the COVID-19 response is justified by the exceptional circumstances of the current pandemic, and their use in this context does not imply that future public health use is ethically appropriate without significant public debate (e.g., use in seasonal flu surveillance efforts). Future use will require independent justification. Use of DCTT in other contexts (e.g., law enforcement or immigration enforcement) is also presumptively unethical.

All in all, the arguments that DCTT should be designed as a minimal system are not convincing. Rather, DCTT should be developed through a "values in design" approach, with a core set of features that protect privacy, with enough flexibility to be used differently depending upon local conditions, evolving evidence, and individual preferences. What kind of digital contact tracing system will strike the right balance between public health goals and other considerations will depend upon circumstances. For example, whether it is even beneficial to provide public health authorities with volumes of data about potential contacts of COV+ people will depend, in part, upon whether they have the capacity to make good use of those data. This will vary from location to location and will change over time.

Recommendations

- Technology companies should not alone control the terms, conditions, or capabilities of DCTT, nor should they presume to know what may be acceptable to members of the public.

- A "values in design" approach to development of DCTT should be adopted (Flanagan, Howe, and Nissenbaum 2008; Knobel and Bowker 2011). Robust public- and user-engagement activities should be pursued to identify and incorporate, to the extent possible, a range of values into the design of the technology. These values may include privacy, but also autonomy, efficiency, equity, or others. Technology design should reflect an appropriate balance and prioritization of identified values.

- Technology design should not be static but rather it should be capable of evolving depending upon local conditions, new evidence, and changing preferences and priorities.

- DCTT should be designed to have a base set of features that protect privacy, with layers of additional capabilities that users may choose to activate. An initial default should be that user location data are not shared, but users should be provided with easy mechanisms and prompts to allow for opting-in to this capability, with encouragement to the public if and as it is shown to be critical to achieving public health goals.

Policy Positions to Advance Widespread
Use of Digital Contact Tracing Technologies

The public health value of a DCTT depends in part on the number of people who use it. This section concerns broad public policy positions that relate to the widespread adoption of DCTT. What are ethical means of encouraging or securing widespread adoption of DCTT systems? Under what circumstances would it be ethical to mandate their use or incentivize their use? What enforcement challenges exist?

Mandating Use

Digital contact tracing has occurred without the public's explicit voluntary agreement in some countries such as China and Israel. In others, use has been voluntary (Valentino-DeVries, Singer, and Krolik 2020). For example, Singapore adopted an app that the public could use on a voluntary basis, and approximately 20% of the population has downloaded and used it. Norway has recently launched a contact tracing app that was downloaded by roughly 30% of the population in the first week that it was made available. In the United States, many advocates and researchers have argued that use of digital contact tracing tools must be fully voluntary; this is the dominant perspective.

There are numerous ways that DCTT could be put into use without user choice. For example, as has been done in Israel, location data from mobile phones could be collected and used by the government without users' consent. Use of an app could be formally mandated as a precondition for returning to work or school, or even further, to control entry into a facility or onto transportation such as airplanes through scanning of a QR code to demonstrate personal exposure levels (Gan and Culver 2020).

While these approaches are hard to imagine in the United States, some contend that mandatory use of digital contact tracing tools could be ethical and may even be ethically required. Mandating use of digital contact tracing tools could, in theory, vastly increase the effectiveness of digital contact tracing systems, and thus may save more lives and allow states to lift lockdowns sooner or avoid reimposing lockdowns in the future. Canca (2020) argues that use of privacy-by-design digital contact tracing tools should be mandatory because the use of these tools will be nearly harmless if there are sufficient privacy protections. In addition, mandatory use of DCTT that embraces these principles is significantly less intrusive at the individual level than manual contact tracing, which involves the collection of personally identifying and potentially sensitive data. In this light, it could be argued that such mandates are actually preferable from the perspective of both public health and individual liberty, insofar as they reduce the likelihood of "stay at home" orders, which are a severe limitation of individual liberty.

Nevertheless, mandated use of DCTT systems faces considerable obstacles. For example, people may not adhere to the mandate by simply leaving their phone at home, thus preventing their activities from being tracked. Even more harmful would be if people react to a mandate and a perceived violation of liberty and privacy by employing location and Bluetooth spoofing software to shield their real contacts behind a screen of misinformation. The introduction of this misinformation into a contact tracing effort might severely undermine its effectiveness. The possibility of nonadherence also raises the issue of enforcement: would high rates of nonadherence be permitted, or would enforcement be attempted (if even possible)? Perhaps more important, should the technology not deliver the hoped-for benefits, having mandated the use of an unproven technology could result in a loss of public trust in the technology, the entity instituting the mandate, and potentially the larger public health response (Bernstein et al. 2019).

Mandatory DCTT could also be used to enforce quarantine restrictions and stay-at-home orders for those who are COV+ or are determined to be at heightened risk. The use of DCTT in enforcement activities raises a number of ethical (and legal) issues that are beyond the scope of the present analysis. In particular, individuals have a heightened interest in personal privacy if their data can be used to restrict their freedom of movement and other civil liberties. At a minimum, stringent procedural protections would be required to ensure that the data collection is fair and unbiased and that DCTT users are provided with adequate information, in advance, about how their data may be used.

Mandatory use policies for DCTT must therefore convincingly address a number of questions, including:

- Is the technology designed to meet an important and unmet public health need?

- Is there sufficient evidence to suggest that the technology will be effective at serving its purpose?

- Is the outbreak characterized by sufficiently severe morbidity and mortality and a high rate of disease transmission?

- Are there other less autonomy-restricting or less risky alternatives to widespread mandatory use of DCTT?

- Is it possible and likely that a sufficient number of individuals will comply with a mandate?

- Can inequities in the burdens and benefits of the mandate be sufficiently addressed through social protections and countermeasures?

- Can enforcement and enforcement discretion be implemented in a manner that is consonant with fundamental rights?

- Will those subject to the mandate interact closely with a population that is at high risk of morbidity or mortality if they contract the virus?

- Is it possible to mandate use and remain consistent with important ethical and legal principles?

These questions would need to be satisfactorily addressed and explicitly documented by any decision maker considering mandatory use, including government officials, institutional leaders, and employers. Particularly important is the need to identify reliable evidence that the DCTT would be effective and to ensure that the burdens and benefits of use are equitable and justifiable. If use of a DCTT is a condition for returning to work or school in person, those who refuse or are unable to use DCTT should not lose their jobs or positions as a result, and adequate support should be in place for people who are asked to self-quarantine.

Finally, it is important to distinguish a mandate from a "pushed" program installation or a default setting in an application which can be modified by users. A mandate relates to a policy of required use, whereas the pushed programs or default settings relate to the chosen architecture for download and operation of the application.

Perhaps the most effective way to generate widespread adoption of DCTT in the United States is to offer incentives to individuals who choose to adopt and who properly utilize the preferred DCTT approach in a voluntary system. External incentives may help "nudge" populations toward desired adoption targets. Given the importance of widespread use of DCTT, modest incentives ought to be considered for DCTT in the US if and when there is sufficient evidence of the technology's utility. Note that in other contexts, studies have shown that the provision of some incentive leads to an increase in adoption or utilization of public health programs (Singer and Ye 2013; Lee et al. 2014). Moreover, even a relatively small incentive can achieve much greater rates of adoption, with some studies demonstrating that the incremental adoption gain decreases as the incentive gets larger (Thornton 2008; Gibson et al. 2019). In the context of COVID-19, incentives that might be both effective and ethically acceptable could include a relatively small monetary token, free or discounted mobile phone service for a period of time, or credit to be used by means of a mobile phone.

Not all incentives are ethically appropriate. For example, making access to lifesaving health care contingent on using a DCTT or making valuable disease information available only to DCTT users would not be ethically appropriate. In addition, incentives cannot be used to overcome otherwise ethically unjustifiable technology design: for example, they should not be used as an offset for providing personally identifiable health information to other users.

Importantly, incentivization schemes must be kept distinct from mandates, as the latter require greater ethical justification. To offer an incentive is to offer something of actual value to individual participants over and above what they are reasonably entitled to at baseline. For example, making a return to work contingent on using DCTT is not offering an incentive but instead imposing a mandate, and it would have to be justified as a mandate.

In the context of COVID-19, it is also necessary to recognize that there is an *inherent* "incentive" behind the technology—that is, the promise of more lives saved, faster pandemic recovery, and the reduction or elimination of blanket physical distancing. Effective public communication of these goals, if and when there is sufficient confidence in the technology, is important.

Encouraging Use

Another important approach to increasing use of DCTT in the United States is for trusted leaders to encourage their use. Community leaders, public figures, health care professionals, and other respected individuals who have the public's trust and goodwill could be enlisted to communicate with the public about DCTT and encourage its use, drawing on notions such as communal responsibility, solidarity, and so on. These encouragements could be combined with other approaches (e.g., small incentives) to optimize reach while continuing to respect individual choice.

Recommendations

- DCTT use should not be mandated at this time given uncertainty about potential harms and benefits. Additional technology, user, and real-world testing is needed.

- Incentives can be a useful complement to encouragements; however, any incentives for users to install and use DCTT must be equitable, should not be coercive, and should align with effective use of the technology (i.e., they should not incentivize downloading an app but then leaving one's phone at home).

- Trusted leaders should be enlisted to communicate effectively with the public about DCTT and encourage its use, should the technology demonstrate some potential. The limits of knowledge regarding effectiveness should also be explained, along with what will be done to improve technological capabilities as understanding evolves.

Disclosure and Authorization/Consent

In deciding whether to use DCTT *voluntarily*, individuals must be sufficiently informed, both through broad coordinated public engagement campaigns and individual-level disclosures, and there must be a meaningful mechanism for users to consent. It is important to recognize that while informed consent—which is characterized by detailed consent forms and requires a witnessed signature—is the standard for most research and clinical care encounters (Faden and Beauchamp 1986), it is not typically the standard for public health disease surveillance. In the public health context, other relevant protections (such ethics training for public health professionals, and strict data handling and confidentiality requirements) are in place and there is a strong public health interest in collecting the relevant data. A more limited role for consent has been recommended for public health surveillance based on a reciprocal obligation of members of society to contribute to a "common good" and, particularly in the context of a pandemic, practical considerations such as time constraints and exigencies such as increasing morbidity and mortality (WHO 2017).*

Under current circumstances, given that (1) many individuals have time and capacity to consent, (2) DCTT is being considered as part of plans for longer-term restabilization, (3) DCTT is not a familiar part of our public lexicon, (4) remote consent disclosure and authorization can be easily embedded in DCTT systems (Moore et al. 2017), and (5) there are justifiable public deficits in trust with respect to various government and corporate actors handling potentially personal digital information, a strong ethical case can be made for requiring a carefully crafted version of what is sometimes referred to as simple consent. Simple consent consists of basic disclosure and voluntary agreement or authorization (Ali et al. 2017). Three questions then arise.

1. **What information should be disclosed to potential users of DCTT?**

   - Information disclosed might include:

     ◦ Entity responsible for the technology

     ◦ Its purpose

     ◦ How it works (in lay terms)

---

* Some participatory disease surveillance systems (e.g., Flu Near You) have received formal "waivers" of consent requirements from institutional review boards (IRBs) in the US. As they undergo development, these digital surveillance systems often straddle a line between public health surveillance and research, hence the frequent need or desire to obtain ethical review by an IRB (Ali et al. 2019).

- What users need to do
- Any user options, e.g.,
    - Sharing geolocation data with public health authorities when that would facilitate a defined public health goal
    - Sharing de-identified metadata with technology developers (for system enhancement)
- User rights
- How data will be handled
    - What data are collected
    - What data are shared (and how and with whom)
    - Purposes for which data can be used and not used
    - How data are secured and protected
    - Whether and what data will be retained (or will be deletable)
- Potential benefits and any known risks
- How to obtain answers to questions about the technology and public health response

2. How should this information be presented?

Information should be presented leveraging eConsent models that are more accessible than long "clickwrap" disclosures typical of mobile apps (Iwaya et al. 2019). For example, a simple open-source smartphone consent module that has been developed by Sage Bionetworks for research uses could be adapted to the public health surveillance context and to DCTT (Doerr, Suver, and Wilbanks 2016).

- Formatting recommendations include (cf. Doerr et al. 2016):
    - simple and straightforward information
    - deliberately organized content
    - multimodal learning (e.g., visual, audio, written)
    - accessibility for disabled users

- ° multilingual text
- ° engagement through interaction (e.g, swiping to navigate forward and backward)

- The same simple information should be made publicly available via multiple other platforms (e.g., on websites, in newspapers, over social media).

- More detailed disclosures should be made readily accessible to those who wish to learn more, with no hidden surprises.

3. How should users signal that they agree to the details specified in disclosures?

Opt-in Models

Opt-in models are those that, through an affirmative act such as clicking a button, users would indicate their intention to use a DCTT. This approach is consistent with other app downloads, where app details and privacy policies are made available through a download page and users are required to affirmatively click a button to install an app. Once installed, some apps further alert users to particular ways in which phone capabilities or data will be used, with some permitting selective toggling (opting-in or opting-out) of certain features. With DCTT apps, in addition to disclosures provided on a download page, the user could be guided through a simple interactive module embedded in the app (such as is described above) in order to increase the chance of meaningful exposure to important information about the technology and how data will be handled. At that point, any user options, such as those itemized above, could be described and choices made.

Opt-out Models

There are at least two different ways in which the term "opt-out" has been used in this context. The conventional use of the term "opt-out" is characterized by an act which signals an individual's intention to decline something that would have otherwise occurred without intervention. A few others have used the term to refer to "revocation of consent," for example, the United States COVID-19 Consumer Data Protection Act of 2020 Senate bill (S.3663) would establish a default opt-in position—

requiring "affirmative express consent" for collection and use of proximity and other related data—and refers to individuals having a right to later revoke their consent through an "opt-out." The latter use of the term is not our focus here.

Given this, a DCTT app that is voluntarily downloaded through an affirmative act would be difficult to characterize as an opt-out approach. This leaves more passive surveillance systems that rely on automatic installation of self-activating technology onto users phones. There are a range of views among the authors of this report about the value of an opt-out approach for DCTT, with some arguing for an opt-out approach on grounds that it might increase coverage and would be ethically acceptable if accompanied by similar disclosures as above to ensure users are aware of the technology and data uses (Mello and Wang 2020). This approach would present users with a mechanism to opt-out if they wish, which should be reasonably easy to effectuate. Under these circumstances, as noted above, an "opt-out" would not be synonymous with mandating use of the technology.

Others among the authors argue that there is reason to believe that opt-in approaches may be able to sufficiently achieve desirable levels of utilization relative to opt-out approaches. Unfortunately, data related to opt-in versus opt-out models of DCTT are very limited. One recent survey (Altmann et al. 2020) found that across five countries (UK, Germany, France, Italy, US), slightly more people reportedly would download an app under an opt-in system (74.8%) than would keep an app on their phone under an opt-out system (67.7%). Moreover, when US respondents were directly asked which approach they would prefer, 60% indicated a preference for opt-in. This remained true across various demographic variables—gender, region, political affiliation, lockdown status, and other characteristics. Whether actual behaviors would align with anticipated behaviors in the context of DCTT remains an unanswered question that should be carefully studied under real-world conditions. There are a range of important empirical questions regarding how much and what kind of impact (positive or negative) various types of defaults might generate for public health and for different mobile phone user groups, including vulnerable and marginalized users.

Opt-out models for app authorization may encounter greater legal and political challenges, especially if the COVID-19 Consumer Data Protection Act of 2020 (S.3663), the competing Public Health Emergency Privacy Act (S.3749), or another similar bill is enacted in the United States. Both of these standing bills require affirmative opt-in consent. Opt-out approaches also risk negative reactions from some mobile phone users, a small number of whom may go so far as to intentionally interfere with data because of the perceived intrusiveness of an automatically installed tracking platform (Dixit 2020).

Given these considerations and the apparent willingness of a large portion of the population to opt-in to use DCTT, an opt-in approach to authorization should be instituted to accompany initial DCTT rollout. The feasibility and value of opt-out approaches should continue to be evaluated, informed by what is technologically possible, what local assessments of benefits and harms of the technology reveal over time, and our evolving understanding of the degree to which an opt-out approach is likely to increase or decrease utilization. Opt-out approaches should not be precluded.

Recommendations

- A clear and concise module consisting of basic disclosure and voluntary authorization should be developed to accompany DCTT. This module should not take the form of "clickwrap" terms of service or end-user agreements but rather provide only essential information necessary for an individual to make a decision. More detailed disclosures (such as FAQs in plain language) should be made easily accessible to those who wish to learn more, with no hidden surprises.

- An opt-in approach to authorization should be instituted to accompany initial DCTT rollout. The feasibility and value of opt-out approaches should continue to be evaluated, informed by what is technologically possible, what local assessments of benefits and harms of the technology reveal over time, and our evolving understanding of the degree to which an opt-out approach is likely to increase or decrease utilization among different populations. Opt-out approaches should not be precluded.

Digital contact tracing technologies should be designed and used in ways that, as far as possible, promote an equitable distribution of benefits and burdens. DCTT should be deployed in a manner that does not propagate preexisting patterns of unfair disadvantage or distribute harms and risks unfairly throughout the population. For example, communities with lower rates of technology and data access may benefit less from DCTT. Special attention must be paid to communities that experience preexisting health disparities and to those that are being hardest hit by the pandemic.

Digital Disparities

In the United States, February 2019 data indicate that approximately 80% of the population are smartphone users (Pew Research Center 2020), though rates of mobile phone use are significantly lower among people over age 65 (53%), people with any disability (58%; 2016 data) (Anderson and Perrin 2017), people with less than a high school education (66%), people who earn less than $30,000 per year (71%), and people who live in rural areas (71%). As a result, these populations and communities may use DCTT in lower numbers, thereby lessening the effectiveness of DCTT and the likelihood of benefit for these populations from such systems. Moreover, it has been reported that many older and less costly smartphones (roughly estimated at 10%–20% of smartphones in the US) lack important capabilities required for the leading Apple/Google platform to work (Bradshaw 2020). This is of special concern because some of the above groups that are less likely to own smartphones in general are also less likely to own newer smartphones with the needed capabilities. Some within the above groups (e.g., people who are older and people identified as Hispanic, African American, or American Indian) are also disproportionately experiencing morbidity and mortality from COVID-19 (CDC 2020h).

One may argue that by using DCTT, human and financial resources that would otherwise be spent on manual contact tracing will be preserved, and these resources can then be redirected to better meet the needs of those who are not otherwise being effectively served by the technology because of disparities or for other reasons. This argument has intuitive appeal and should be taken seriously; however, it is unsettled whether DCTT will contribute sufficient efficiencies to the overall public health response to make it possible, financially and logistically, for manual services to be allocated in greater proportion to those who are unable to benefit from DCTT. It is entirely possible that, at least in the short-term, DCTT may introduce new inefficiencies due to unintended consequences or the need for public health officials to follow up many more contacts. One possible mitigation to the challenge of digital disparity—though it does not solve the underlying challenge of ensuring net efficiency across systems—might be to provide mobile phones or other devices and data packages to those who would otherwise be left out.

Disparate Risk of Harm from Surveillance and Data Gathering

Ensuring wide digital coverage does not, however, resolve other equity concerns. It is important to consider that some populations may experience greater harm, and fear of harm, from having their data collected. For example, some groups such as African Americans, Hispanic Americans, Muslim Americans, and undocumented immigrants have more reasonable fear of their data being handed over to law or immigration enforcement, and some groups have lower levels of trust in public health due to past injustices (CSM 2017; Pew Research Center 2017; Rodrigues et al. 2018; Auxier et al. 2019). Any data gathered by DCTT should be used solely for public health purposes. Efforts should be made to assure members of these and other communities that their data will not be misused or made available to those outside of a public health context. In addition, if DCTT are used in the current pandemic, this should be with the understanding that future use of DCTT in other contexts (e.g., law enforcement or immigration enforcement) is presumptively unethical.

Some preliminary polling related specifically to DCTT emphasizes the complexity of the challenges faced and the need for deeper public engagement (Anderson and Auxier 2020). The polling results suggest that people who identify as African American or Hispanic are more likely than people who identify as White to consider government tracking of mobile phones as acceptable. These findings, like many others, are difficult to interpret given background political polarization on the issue. More direct engagement is required to better understand how different communities comprehend and experience DCTT and other forms of surveillance.

Discrimination and Stigma

Stigma may result from an individual being identified as COV+, or a neighborhood or establishment becoming identified as a "hotspot" as a result of numerous COV+ people living in that area or having visited that establishment. In particular, certain groups may suffer more as a result of being associated with COVID-19, such as the well-documented blame that has been directed toward Chinese people (and broadly East Asian communities) or the communities that are disproportionately likely to contract the illness (Devakumar et al. 2020). When identifiable location data are made public, as has been the case in South Korea, personal and private information were revealed. Furthermore, businesses in South Korea that were identified as having patrons who tested positive for COVID-19 have suffered economic losses and stigma (N. Kim 2020).

To avoid the stigma and potential discrimination that can result from being identified as COV+, DCTT must never make data publicly available that could be used to identify persons who have tested positive. Safeguards must be in place to ensure that any identifiable data that may be gathered for public health purposes are protected. If DCTT data are used to provide heat maps to the public of locations that COV+ individuals frequently visit so as to provide representations of geographic risk or for other reasons, it is essential that care be taken to avoid unfairly distributing further economic burdens or other stigmatizing and discriminatory outcomes.

Recommendations

- A commitment to equity means a commitment to ensuring that the benefits and burdens of DCTT are distributed fairly. Public engagement is an important tool for assessing impact and to rectify inequities.

- States, localities, and institutions that recommend widespread use of DCTT should provide technology (e.g., mobile phones, Bluetooth devices) and free data packages to those who desire but lack access to these devices.

- If there are lower rates of adoption of DCTT systems in some identifiable communities, public health authorities should identify ways to compensate. For example, directing more non-DCTT resources and efforts toward those communities to meet specific needs that are elsewhere being supported by technology.

- If maps are generated based on DCTT to provide the public with the locations that COV+ individuals have visited, steps must be taken to minimize the stigma and potential financial losses that could result from being identified as a hotspot.

Instituting Transparent Governance and Oversight

DCTT must be developed with an eye toward both present and future implications. Transparent and publicly trustworthy management, governance, and oversight of DCTT technology and data is both a near- and long-term necessity. We face significant uncertainties. DCTT technologies are rapidly developing. Their risks, capabilities, effectiveness, and downstream implications are not yet well understood.

Concerns about "Surveillance Creep"

Significant concerns have been expressed by privacy advocates (Guariglia 2020) and in the popular press (Giglio 2020) about what is known as "surveillance creep." Their worry is that state and corporate actors will use new surveillance technologies, capacities, and permissions well beyond the purposes for which they were initially justified to the public and beyond the time when they are useful for the COVID-19 pandemic.

Surveillance creep should be guarded against. Only those data that are necessary and relevant for the public health purposes at hand should be collected and used, and data should be kept only for the period of time needed for those public health purposes. Data should be used only for public health purposes.

Any use of DCTT during the current pandemic would be justified by the circumstances of this pandemic, and its use in this context does not set a precedent for future public health use (e.g., use in seasonal flu surveillance efforts). Future use will require independent justification. Use of DCTT in the future in other contexts (e.g., law enforcement or immigration enforcement) is presumptively unethical.

Broadly speaking, efforts should be made to generate public awareness and consensus that use of DCTT in COVID-19 efforts does not imply that future use is justifiable. However, generating this public awareness may be particularly challenging given the complexity of the informational environment, where public debate ranges from legitimate concerns about surveillance creep to conspiracy theories regarding the origins of the COVID-19 pandemic (Muller 2020). This means authorities bear special obligations to be clear on how they plan to use the technologies, what oversight mechanisms will be employed to address potential abuse, and how they intend to publicize the conditions under which programs will be terminated, making sure they are followed.

Oversight and Ethical Review

We are rapidly gaining knowledge about SARS-CoV-2 and COVID-19, but we still have essential gaps in our understanding. In the United States, public health responses including DCTT will generally be developed and coordinated by individual states, regional consortia, and associations (Reston, Sgueglia, and Mossburg 2020). Good governance in this context requires transparency and the creation of oversight bodies with the appropriate expertise and representation to allow nimble and effective responses while serving as trusted representatives.

To address the range of ethics-related concerns about the design and use of DCTT, digital surveillance oversight committees should be established, perhaps at a state level and with a platform for national coordination. These committees can provide ethical and regulatory review prior to and concurrent with widespread use of DCTT. These committees should be composed of a diverse group of experts capable of evaluating a DCTT system locally, including members of communities that experience higher rates of digital disparity.

When assessing the design and use of digital contact tracing systems, these committees (and the public more widely) should consider not only the risks and benefits accrued during the COVID-19 pandemic but also implications for the future. What kind of precedent might use of these technologies during the current pandemic set for future use capabilities in other infectious disease outbreaks or in other social contexts (e.g., law enforcement)? How can we navigate safe use of these technologies in a way that preserves public trust in them and enables the possibility of future beneficial use?

As a start, it should be emphasized that principles offered in this and other guidance documents do not apply only during the pandemic. Future efforts to advance DCTT capabilities, during quieter times, should make every effort to follow them.

Recommendations

- Digital surveillance oversight committees should be established expeditiously, with diverse and qualified membership, to provide ethical and regulatory review prior to and concurrent with widespread use of a DCTT system.

- Understandable and publicly accessible rules must guide the collection, access, control, use, storage, and combination of data by government authorities, public and private institutions, and other parties such as public health researchers.

- Only those data that are necessary and relevant for the public health response to COVID-19 should be collected and used.

- Identifiable data should be kept only for the period of time needed for the public health response to COVID-19.

- Identifiable data collected as part of this response should not be shared with anyone other than the relevant public health authorities without additional specific informed consent of individual users.

- Before a government or institution adopts a digital contact tracing program, they should state the conditions under which the digital contact tracing program will be terminated.

- Future use of DCTT to advance public health or other efforts (e.g., use in seasonal flu surveillance) would require independent justification. DCTT designed for public health use should not be used by law or immigration enforcement.

- The principles offered in this guidance document apply both during and following the COVID-19 pandemic.

FOUR

Legal Considerations

The implementation of digital contact tracing technology (DCTT) is likely to implicate a number of US laws at both the federal and state levels. This section focuses primarily on federal laws, as these laws apply nationwide and generally preempt conflicting state laws. A comprehensive assessment of the legality of any particular DCTT program would require case-specific analysis and attention to relevant state laws, including any that specifically address DCTT, which may soon exist in one or more states. The analysis here is limited to the United States; foreign and international laws will not be addressed.

Many of the laws discussed in this section are privacy laws designed to protect individuals from the harms that may result from the unauthorized or improper use of their personally identifiable information (PII). Under these laws, legal concerns will generally be minimized if privacy protections are built directly into the DCTT technology (e.g., "privacy by design"). As a general principle, DCTT should be designed to collect and store only as much PII as is necessary to achieve the public health purpose. Collecting only proximity data, for example, is likely to raise fewer legal concerns than collecting both proximity data and geolocation data. Likewise, creating aggregated, anonymized, or de-identified data will raise fewer legal concerns than using and disclosing PII.

As we have argued elsewhere in this guidance document, however, the public health and societal crisis caused by COVID-19 may justify greater encroachments on individual privacy than would otherwise be permissible. Regardless of the type of data collected, privacy concerns will be reduced if users are afforded the right to choose whether their PII is collected and how it is used and disclosed. As such, DCTT should generally secure meaningful user consent before collecting PII, a process which typically requires both disclosure of relevant information and agreement on the part of the user.

Privacy concerns will also be reduced if the use of PII is strictly limited to tracking and limiting the spread of SARS-CoV-2. The use of DCTT data for other purposes—such as commercial or law enforcement purposes—would raise additional legal and ethical concerns. In addition, DCTT developers may be required to implement governance policies that ensure the secure storage of PII, limit data retention periods, require transparency about data sharing, and maintain records of responses to data requests from government authorities.

In short, the legality of a DCTT program under current United States law will depend on a number of factors, including what type of data is collected; how the data are used and who may access them; how user consent is obtained; whether the entity collecting and using the data is the government or a private corporation; the context in which data are collected (e.g., employment, education, or commercial); and which states have jurisdiction over the program.

Privacy law in the United States, unlike in other jurisdictions such as the European Union (EU) and Australia, is generally sector-specific and limited in scope. The result is a patchwork of protections that differ significantly depending on the entity that collects the data and the type of data collected. For example, under current law, telecommunication carriers are governed by different privacy rules than mobile broadband providers. Given the complexity of existing federal privacy law, we believe that it would be beneficial for the US Congress to enact new privacy legislation that is specifically tailored to the use of DCTT in response to COVID-19. Congress appears poised at least to debate such legislation: a pair of bills recently introduced in the Senate and one in the House of Representatives would significantly restrict the collection of PII by digital devices for COVID-tracing purposes. S.3663, S.3749, H.R. 6866, 116th Cong. (2020).

Telecommunications

A DCTT provider that collects data from a user's mobile phone may be subject to the privacy rules governing telecommunication carriers, which are enforced by the Federal Communications Commission (FCC). The data protected under these rules are limited, however, to certain types of PII, termed "customer proprietary network information" (CPNI). Moreover, the rules generally apply only to telecommunications carriers and interconnected VoIP (Voice over Internet Protocol) providers.

In particular, under section 222 of the Communications Act of 1934, 47 U.S.C. § 222, and the implementing regulations of the Federal Communications Commission (FCC), telecommunications carriers and VoIP providers must establish and maintain systems designed to ensure that they adequately protect their subscribers' CPNI, and they are generally restricted from using or disclosing CPNI without the customer's consent (unless the use of disclosure is needed to provide the services subscribed to by the customer). If customer consent is sought to use or disclose CPNI, individual notice must be provided to the customer, and such notice must provide sufficient information to enable the customer to make an informed decision as to whether to permit the requested use or disclosure.

CPNI is individually identifiable information that carriers and providers have collected about their customers, including phone numbers called and the frequency, duration, and timing of such calls. Of most relevance to DCTT, a recent FCC Notice of Apparent Liability asserted that user geolocation data collected by mobile phone network carriers qualify as CPNI under § 222 and related rules. 35 FCC Rcd 1785 (2) (2020). Pursuant to this notice, the FCC fined T-Mobile for selling to third parties location data that were derived from the communication between the mobile phones of T-Mobile's customers and nearby network signal towers. (The FCC also levied fines against AT&T, Verizon, and Sprint on the same grounds (Valentino-DeVries 2020).) While the FCC has made its position clear that geolocation data are CPNI, courts have yet to weigh in on the matter.

Even if geolocation data are CPNI, however, the FCC can enforce § 222 of the Communications Act only against telecom carriers and VoIP providers, not against cable broadband and mobile broadband internet providers. 47 U.S.C. § 53(44), 47 C.F.R. § 9.3. In 2018, the FCC promulgated a regulation stating that, contrary to its prior position, its § 222 authority does not extend to cable broadband and mobile broadband internet providers. Restoring Internet Freedom, 83 Fed. Reg. 7852 (Feb. 2, 2020) (to be codified at 47 C.F.R. pts. 1, 8, and 20). This regulatory shift was subsequently upheld by the DC Circuit, *Mozilla Corporation v. Federal Communications Commission*, 940 F.3d 1 (2019).

In addition to § 222, the FCC has authority to regulate "common carriers"—including both telecommunication carriers and broadband internet providers—under § 201(b) of the Communications Act. In the past, the FCC has interpreted § 201(b) to protect against "unjust and unreasonable" privacy and data security practices with respect to customers' personal information beyond CPNI. In 2016, the FCC promulgated a regulation asserting its authority under this interpretation. However, Congress overturned this regulation pursuant to the Congressional Review Act in 2017. S.J. Res. 34, 115th Cong. (2017). At present, the extent of the FCC's authority under § 201(b) remains unsettled (Mulligan and Linebaugh 2019).

Consumer Protection

The collection, storage, release, and transmission of digital user data, including proximity contacts, is more generally governed by the Federal Trade Commission (FTC). The FTC is an independent US law enforcement agency tasked with protecting consumers and promoting competition across broad sectors of the economy (FTC 2020). The FTC's primary legal authority with respect to consumer protection comes from Section 5 of the FTC Act, which prohibits "unfair or deceptive acts or practices in or affecting commerce." 15 U.S.C. § 45(a)(1). Note that the FTC and FCC have some overlapping authority to protect consumer privacy in the context of telecommunications (FCC and FTC 2017).

The FTC has interpreted Section 5 to require companies to be transparent and accurate about their collection of PII from consumers. A company may be found to have engaged in a deceptive practice if it fails to disclose that it is collecting user data or fails to disclose that it is sharing these data with third parties and to provide a general description of these third parties. The FTC has used its authority under Section 5 numerous times to discipline companies that purport in published privacy policies or other notices to provide protection for the privacy and/or security of personal information, yet fail to do so in practice. For example, the FTC may find it both "unfair" and "deceptive" for a mobile app privacy policy to state that the app never discloses location information to third parties, when in fact the app shares that information with the app developer's service provider, which in turn uses it to provide analytical data to the app developer that are used to create targeted advertising.

The FTC does not use its Section 5 authority other than to protect consumers and generally does not consider "de-identified" user data, which are data that are not "reasonably linkable" to a consumer, to be a subject for consumer protection. In general, data collected are not "reasonably linkable" so long as the company collecting it "(1) takes reasonable measures to ensure that the data are de-identified; (2) publicly commits not to try to reidentify the data; and (3) contractually prohibits downstream recipients from trying to reidentify the data" (FTC 2012).

Many states have laws that are similar to Section 5, prohibiting unfair and deceptive acts and practices. Both Section 5 and these similar state laws can be violated not only by misrepresentations (affirmative deception) but also by material omissions. Thus, a failure to inform an app user of the app's collection of tracking data and the planned use and disclosure of those data could constitute a violation of these laws. Companies providing DCTT apps should make sure that all such information is disclosed in the apps' terms of use to which users must affirmatively agree.

Children's Online Privacy

Children who use DCTT may be protected by additional privacy protections. In particular, collection of digital PII from children under the age of 13 is strictly regulated under the Children's Online Privacy Protection Act (COPPA) (15 U.S.C. §§ 6501–6505). Under COPPA, PII includes "first and last name[;] a persistent identifier that can be used to recognize a user over time and across different . . . online services[;] and geolocation information sufficient to identify street name and name of a city or town[.]" COPPA prohibits a website or online service from collecting personal information (including location information) from children under age 13 without obtaining verifiable parental consent. Note that there may be an exception to this requirement for an "investigation on a matter related to public safety." 16 CFR § 312.5(c)(6)(iv).

Electronic Surveillance

In addition to misuse of user data by DCTT providers, another privacy concern is that a third party may be able to access sensitive PII that is collected and stored by a DCTT system without the user's knowledge and consent. There are a number of federal criminal laws, however, that would likely prohibit such unauthorized access to PII.

In particular, the Electronic Communications Privacy Act of 1986 (ECPA)—which includes the Wiretap Act (18 U.S.C. §§ 2510–2522), the Stored Communications Act (18 U.S.C. §§ 2701–2711), and the Pen Register Act (18 U.S.C. §§ 3121–3127)—makes it a crime to access electronic communications without authorization. Individuals who violate the ECPA face up to five years in prison and fines up to $250,000. Victims are also entitled to bring civil suits and recover actual damages, in addition to punitive damages and attorney's fees, for violations.

Generally, the access restrictions in the ECPA apply unless consent is given or if access is authorized by statute for law enforcement purposes. For example, an employer is generally forbidden from accessing an employee's private emails. However, if consent is given in the form of an employment contract that explicitly authorizes the employer to access emails, it may be lawful under the ECPA for the employer to access such information. Along the same lines, the ECPA would likely prohibit an employer from accessing contact tracing data on an employee's phone without the employee's consent. However, the ECPA would likely not prohibit duly authorized government public health officials from accessing contact tracing data without consent.

As its name suggests, the Stored Communications Act (SCA) regulates access to communications at rest, that is, not in transit. The SCA makes it unlawful to intentionally access a facility in which electronic communication services are provided and to obtain, alter, or prevent authorized access to a wire or electronic communication while it is in electronic storage in such a system. As such, the SCA would likely apply only to centralized collection of contact tracing data.

The Pen Register Act covers any "signaling information" exchanged in a communication, such as phone numbers. The statute does not reach the content of such communications, however. An expansive interpretation of the Pen Register Act would cover Bluetooth "handshakes," as they are merely signaling information between devices, which do not carry content. See *United States v. Forrester,* 512 F.3d 500 (9th Cir. 2007) (finding that email headers and IP addresses are akin to pen registers and have no Fourth Amendment protection). Unlike the SCA, there is no statutory exclusionary rule that applies when the government illegally uses a pen register / trap and trace device. Additionally, there is no private cause of action against the government for violations of the Pen Register Act.

State Data Privacy Laws

States have a variety of privacy laws and are increasingly seeking to regulate the online collection of personal information and the use and disclosure of such information. To date, most of these laws focus more on transparency and protection from unauthorized access than on restricted collection and use (except with respect to biometric information), seeking to ensure that individuals who use websites or online services such as mobile applications do so on an informed basis with respect to the privacy provided by those sites and services. Two examples of such state laws are the California Online Privacy Protection Act (CalOPPA) and the California Consumer Privacy Act (CCPA). Both laws require notice to individuals who use websites or online services such as mobile applications, in order to ensure that users are informed about the privacy of personal information collected by those sites and services. (The CCPA also applies to data collection off-line.) Both laws treat IP addresses and location data as types of potentially identifiable personal data, and so would very likely apply to DCTT apps used by California residents.

CalOPPA requires that the operator of any website, mobile application, or other online service ("Site") post a privacy policy on the Site disclosing certain information regarding the Site's collection, use, and disclosure of PII. CalOPPA applies to any Site that is accessible to California residents. The required disclosures are not onerous and would apply only to collection of data that are identifiable to an individual person (but, depending on who collects the data, location data together with a device identifier are identifiable to the user).

The CCPA requires that any entity qualifying as a "business" provide its "consumers"—defined as lawful residents of California—with specific disclosures about the business's collection, use, and disclosure of personal information. Importantly, the CCPA applies only to for-profit businesses that meet certain thresholds of revenue or access to consumer information. A public health agency or a nonprofit organization would not be subject to the CCPA. Cal. Civ. Code § 1798.140(c).

The CCPA defines "personal information" as "information that identifies, relates to, describes, is reasonably capable of being associated with, or could reasonably be linked, directly or indirectly, with a particular consumer or household." The statute provides a nonexclusive list of potential identifiable personal information, including "geolocation data." In accordance with the CCPA, businesses must provide consumers with a notice "at or before the point of collection" of personal information, which must describe the personal information to be collected and the purposes for collecting that information. Businesses must additionally allow consumers to request access to and request deletion of personal information. Businesses must allow for consumers to opt-out of the sale of any personal information. Developers of COVID-tracing apps would want to build in compliance with these requirements. In addition, California Civil Code § 1798.81.5(a)(1) requires companies to "maintain reasonable security procedures and practices appropriate to the nature of the information it processes."

Like privacy laws generally, the CCPA does not grant consumers rights regarding the use of de-identified information. However, the CCPA does require businesses to implement processes that prohibit re-identification of de-identified information, as well as technical safeguards to prevent inadvertent release of that information. Cal. Civ. Code § 1798.140(h).

Health Information Privacy

Many DCTT systems will be designed to collect health-related data of users, such as symptom tracking, SARS-CoV-2 test results, and prior exposure to a person who is COV+. Individuals may have additional privacy protections with respect to the use and disclosure of this health-related information.

The use and disclosure of individually identifiable health information is strictly regulated under the privacy and security rules implementing the

Health Insurance Portability and Accountability Act (HIPAA). HIPAA is limited in application, however, to health care providers and health insurance plans ("covered entities") and "business associates" of such entities. "Business associates" under HIPAA are persons who perform services for covered entities and need access to personal health information to do so.

HIPAA-covered entities must have written authorization to use or disclose identifiable health information ("protected health information," or PHI) from the individual to whom such information pertains, unless the HIPAA regulations promulgated by the US Department of Health and Human Services (HHS) provide an exception to the requirement for such individual authorization.

Among the exceptions to the individual authorization requirement is an exception for certain uses and disclosures of PHI for public health purposes. 45 CFR § 164.512(b). This exception would permit, for example, a HIPAA-covered entity to disclose the PHI of an individual who tests positive for SARS-CoV-2 to a public health authority. A "public health authority" is an agency or authority of the US government, a state, territory, a political subdivision of a state or territory, or Indian tribe that is responsible for public health matters as part of its official mandate, as well as a person or entity acting under a grant of authority from, or under a contract with, a public health agency, such as a contact tracer. Id. § 164.501.

Many DCTT developers are HIPAA business associates, and any use and disclosure of PHI collected through DCTT used on behalf of HIPAA-covered entities is restricted under the HIPAA privacy rules. Notably, in response to COVID-19, HHS announced that its Office for Civil Rights would exercise its enforcement discretion and would not impose penalties for violations of certain provisions of the HIPAA Privacy Rule against health care providers or their business associates for the good faith uses and disclosures of protected health information for public health and health oversight activities during the nationwide public health emergency. 85 FR 19392 (2020).

Many states also have health information privacy laws. The HIPAA privacy rule sets a "floor" of privacy protections, allowing the states to be more protective of privacy. More specifically, HIPAA preempts a state law if (but only if) the state law is "contrary" and less protective of privacy than the HIPAA privacy rule. However, if a state law is determined by the

Secretary of HSS to be necessary to serve a "compelling need related to public health, safety, or welfare," it may survive preemption even if it is less privacy-protective than HIPAA. 45 CFR § 160.203 (a)(1)(iv).

The Public Health Service Act also restricts the use of certain personally identifiable information collected by entities involved with public health activities without the individual's consent. 42 U.S.C. 242m(d).

Labor and Employment Privacy Rights

Labor and employment laws—that is, laws that govern the relationships between employers and employees—may prove relevant to DCTT, especially if employers mandate the use of DCTT or seek to collect health information regarding their employees using DCTT. Depending on the built-in privacy protections of the DCTT system, an employer may be able to access important health information from an employee's phone. As noted above, the ECPA would generally prohibit an employer from accessing this information without the employee's consent. Even with consent, however, there are limits on the collection and use of an employee's health information.

In particular, the use of DCTT may raise special concerns about employment discrimination, for example, if an employer were to fire an employee who tests positive for SARS-CoV-2 (COV+) or who has a known SARS-CoV-2 exposure. The Americans with Disabilities Act (ADA) protects disabled employees from discrimination and restricts the collection of personal health information by employers. The Equal Employment Opportunity Commission (EEOC), which is the federal agency tasked with enforcing the ADA in the employment context, would likely consider COV+ to be a "disability" under the ADA and analogous state laws prohibiting discrimination against disabled people. COV+ is likely to be a "disability," especially where the individual is symptomatic and/or experiences related health issues, or if it is later determined that testing positive for SARS-CoV-2 leads to long-term or chronic health effects. "Exposure to a COV+ person" could also be covered by those laws because a person exposed to a COV+ individual could well be perceived as being disabled by being considered likely to be infected.

The ADA generally requires that businesses make "reasonable accommodations" for persons who are disabled, which may include individuals who are COV+ or who have a preexisting disability that places them at higher risk from or may be exacerbated by COVID-19. The EEOC has published guidance on reasonable accommodations under the ADA and related laws in the context of COVID-19 (EEOC 2020). Among other things, this guidance clarifies that, consistent with the ADA, employers may take temperatures or otherwise collect health information about employees during the pandemic crisis, so long as they keep that information confidential. As of May 18, 2020, the EEOC has not provided guidance that specifically addresses the applicability of the ADA to the use of DCTT by employers.

In addition, employment laws, such as the ADA and the Family and Medical Leave Act (FMLA), and state law equivalents, generally limit disclosure of information and require employers to keep confidential any employee personal health information related to a disability or request for medical leave. Under the ADA, any information regarding the medical condition or history of an employee that an employer obtains as part of an examination or inquiry into a disability could constitute a confidential medical record that can be disclosed only to certain individuals in limited circumstances. 42 U.S.C. §§ 12112(d)(3)(B) and 12112(d)(4). The FMLA also prevents the disclosure of records related to medical histories in connection with an employee's leave request or eligibility. 29 C.F.R. § 825.500(g). The EEOC and some courts have gone further and taken the position that any information concerning an employee's medical condition is protected under the ADA or FMLA.

As discussed elsewhere in this guidance document, employers may have a good reason to employ DCTT in order to ensure workplace safety and limit the spread of SARS-CoV-2 in the community. Employers may also face legal liability if they fail to protect employees (or customers) from potential exposure or infection. In particular, employers have an obligation under the Occupational Safety and Health Act to keep the workplace safe for employees. In response to COVID-19, the Occupational Safety and Health Administration (OSHA) has developed guidance on preparing the workplace (OSHA 2020). The CDC has also prepared guidance on healthy business operations and reducing the spread of SARS-CoV-2 in the workplace (CDC 2020c). Employers must strike an appropriate balance between avoiding employment discrimination and promoting workplace safety.

Reflecting the need for such a balance, the employee protections under the ADA and other employment laws are not absolute and are limited by, among other things, the need to protect the health and safety of other employees and the public. Protection for workplace safety and health generally will justify appropriately tailored measures, such as inquiries into an employee's personal health status or whether someone has tested positive for SARS-CoV-2, temperature checks, and removal of employees from the workplace who are experiencing symptoms or have tested positive and have not been cleared to return to work.

Note, finally, that the use of DCTT by employers should be evaluated in conjunction with the hazard pay, sick leave, and other benefits that are available to employees. Under the Families First Coronavirus Response Act, employers with more than 50 employees and fewer than 500 employees are required to provide two weeks of paid sick leave to an employee who stays home because of COVID-19. Pub. L. No. 116-127, 134 Stat. 178 (2020). This paid leave extends to those who are themselves ill, are quarantined, or are awaiting a diagnosis, as well as those who are caring for sick family members. However, reporting suggests that more than 75% of US workers will not qualify for benefits under this act (Cochrane, Miller, and Tankersley 2020).

Constitutional Privacy Rights

A DCTT program involving only private actors operating on the basis of voluntarily provided information would not present constitutional privacy issues. But any government-directed use of digital technology to support public health tracking and contact tracing involving mandatory government surveillance may potentially implicate a variety of constitutional protections. These constitutional protections apply to actions taken by any level of government in the United States. While state governments have broad policing powers in the area of public health (*Jacobson v. Massachusetts*, 197 U.S. 11 (1905)), and are generally allowed to enforce legislation not preempted by federal laws, even emergency and health-protective laws must be consistent with the US Constitution (HHS 2019; CDC 2020f).

Fourth Amendment Search and Seizure

Many people considering whether to use a DCTT app may be concerned that government enforcement agencies would obtain tracing data and use those data to conduct criminal prosecutions or immigration proceedings. Constitutional protections, notably the Fourth Amendment's limit on warrantless searches, limit the government's use of personal data in the criminal context. However, exceptions exist, allowing law enforcement to access information even when such access would generally be prohibited. How the government accesses personal data stemming from contact tracing needs to be scrutinized, and protections will hinge on the manner of access.

In general, the Fourth Amendment protects "[t]he right of the people to be secure in their persons, houses, papers, and effects, against unreasonable searches and seizures." As originally interpreted, the Fourth Amendment was considered tied to common-law trespass. That is no longer the case. US Supreme Court precedent interprets the Fourth Amendment to protect "people, not places" and extends to the protection of certain expectations of privacy, such as location information, as long as such expectations are reasonable. *Katz v. United States*, 389 U.S. 347, 351 (1967). A warrantless government search is unconstitutional when the information sought is private and such expectation of privacy is "one that society is prepared to recognize as reasonable." *Smith v. Maryland*, 442 U.S. 735, 743–44 (1979).

The constitutionality of a search will revolve around the following analysis: whether the digital program either violates an individual's "reasonable expectation of privacy" (likely triggered by programs collecting large amounts of location and/or health data) or involves a government "trespass" (likely triggered by required app downloads). *Katz v. United States*, 389 U.S. 347 (1967), *United States v. Jones*, 565 U.S. 400 (2012).

Courts will most likely weigh the intrusiveness of the measures taken in implementing a search standard against the severity of the situation, governmental and individual interests, and accountability measures and safeguards built into the system.

Voluntary sharing by individuals of their information with other parties, including the government, would mean that there was no reasonable expectation of privacy and would not raise the issues elaborated above. It is worth noting that consent may not be considered voluntary if coerced or conditioned, especially with regard to public employees or students of public institutions.

Third-Party Doctrine

Some legal doctrines allow for the government's acquisition of otherwise private information consistent with Fourth Amendment privacy protections. The third-party doctrine, for example, provides that individuals have no reasonable expectation of privacy in information voluntarily shared with others, even if the information is revealed on the assumption that it will be used only for a limited purpose and the confidence placed in the third party will not be betrayed. *Smith v. Maryland*, 442 U.S. 735 (1979), *United States v. Miller*, 425 U.S. 435 (1976). This applies to information provided by third parties (mobile carriers, internet service providers, medical tracking device manufacturers, etc.) to the government under order or request, even when the third party's end-user agreements or privacy policies create an expectation of privacy.

The Supreme Court has narrowed the applicability of the third-party doctrine to exclude use and disclosure of "historical" cell-site location information (CSLI) data. For example, in *Carpenter v. United States*, 138 S. Ct. 2206 (2018), the Court reasoned that the third-party doctrine does not justify use and disclosure of historical CSLI because an individual does not provide that information voluntarily. Rather, that information is pervasively collected by the cell phone company without any affirmative action on the part of the individual. The Court did not express a view on "real-time" CSLI—location information that live-tracks a cell phone's location—or on GPS data that may be stored in the phone itself.

The Carpenter decision builds on a line of cases related to searches of digitally stored location data. In *Riley v. California*, 134 S. Ct. 2473 (2014), the Court held that absent exigent circumstances, law enforcement must obtain a warrant to search an individual's phone. Exigent circumstances are those that require immediate action because there is a probability that evidence may be destroyed. The use of a centralized database for collection of digital contact tracing data would obviate deletion concerns. If the data are stored locally in the phone, issues may arise as to whether law enforcement may suspect the data may be deleted following an arrest.

Similarly, in *United States v. Jones*, 132 S. Ct. 945 (2012), Justice Sonia Sotomayor authored a concurring opinion, arguing that the use of a GPS to track a defendant's whereabouts has the potential of providing the government with enough data points to create a "mosaic" of the person's life. Location data obtained through centralized location contact tracing have the potential of providing information on an individual's whereabouts beyond what's necessary for determining proximity to infected individuals. Localized data may also raise the same issues if accessed by law enforcement.

Following *Carpenter*, several courts have addressed the constitutionality of novel location tracking. In Massachusetts, for instance, a federal district court concluded that police use of a "pole camera" on a utility pole to investigate the movements of an individual constituted a search under the Fourth Amendment. *United States v. Moore-Bush*, 381 F.Supp.3d 139 (D. Mass. 2019). The court reasoned that, even in a public space, an individual still retains a reasonable expectation of privacy "in the whole of their physical movements." Citing *Carpenter* and *Jones*, the court stated that the government's unrestrained power to collect data that reveal private aspects of identity is susceptible to abuse and gives police access to a category of information that is "otherwise unknowable." Long-term monitoring of a person's movements, consequently, violates that individual's expectation of privacy. Notably, the court emphasized the capability of the camera to create a searchable digital log of the photos taken for the eight-month period during which the camera was used.

State courts have also weighed in on the issue. The Massachusetts Supreme Judicial Court found that police access to real-time location data pinpointing an individual's movement, whether from a third party or a cell-site simulator, infringes upon an individual's reasonable expectation of privacy. *Commonwealth v. Almonor*, 120 N.E.3d 1183, 1195 (Mass. 2019). The Washington Supreme Court, for its part, held that a cell phone ping used to locate the defendant's vehicle in real time is a search under the Fourth Amendment requiring a warrant absent exigent circumstances. *State v. Muhammad*, 428 P.3d 1177 (2018). And the Colorado Court of Appeals held that police use of a video pole camera to continuously surveil a defendant's fenced-in backyard constitutes a search under the Fourth Amendment. *People v. Tafoya*, 2019 BL 457321, Colo. Ct. App., 17CA1243 (2019).

Application of *Carpenter* by lower courts to novel location-tracking tactics is still evolving, and it is as yet unclear how the narrower interpretation of the third-party doctrine will continue to be expanded and applied, particularly in cases of short-term monitoring of massive amounts of location and/or health data. Moreover, it is unclear whether *Carpenter* would apply to DCTT data collected by the government itself.

Special Needs Doctrine

An argument in favor of the constitutionality of government DCTT programs is that the "special needs" doctrine would apply. Under this doctrine, a warrantless search that would otherwise violate the Fourth Amendment might be permissible based on a special need relating to public health. When the search is conducted for a nontraditional law enforcement purpose, and circumstances make securing a warrant impracticable, the Supreme Court has ruled that warrantless searches may be permissible. The special needs doctrine, however, is highly controversial because it is not a consistently applied Fourth Amendment exception, so it is difficult to predict when courts would authorize nontraditional surveillance. Some factors considered by the court are (1) the balance between the intrusiveness of the government action and the anticipated public benefits, (2) the existence of legislative authorization, (3) judicial process or the ability of the subject individual to challenge the government action, (4) the scope or breadth of government action, and (5) the likelihood of the collected data being used in criminal proceedings. The Supreme Court did note in *Chandler v. Miller*, 520 U.S. 305 (1997), that a "risk to public safety [that] is substantial and real" may justify "blanket suspicionless searches calibrated to the risk," citing as examples the routine searches conducted at airports and entrances to some official buildings. (Searches within the context of immigration are further analyzed below.)

Immigration Enforcement

Exceptions apply to the constitutional requirement that a warrant accompany an unreasonable search or seizure in the immigration context.

For example, an exception to the general warrant requirement is the border search exception, which allows government officials to search and seize, without a warrant, persons and property at the border or at the functional equivalent of a border. See *United States v. Montoya de Hernandez*, 473 U.S. 531 (1985); *United States v. Flores-Montano*, 541 U.S. 149 (2004). Federal regulation authorizes immigration officials to operate within 100 miles of any US external boundary. (See 8 CFR § 287.1, defining "reasonable distance" as "within 100 air miles from any external boundary of the United States.") A functional equivalent of a border may include any airport where international flights may be received, automobile checkpoints servicing international traffic, and vessels in territorial waters. Government officials, however, must still have "reasonable suspicion" of an immigration violation or a crime to search or seize persons or property.

In the context of digital data, Customs and Border Protection (CBP) officials may conduct either manual or forensic searches of electronic devices at the border, or its functional equivalent. A manual search is considered a routine search and may include accessing the phone and "browsing" its contents. If the electronic device is password protected, individuals must provide information for unlocking the device. Forensic searches, on the other hand, are nonroutine and involve a more invasive search of the electronic device's contents. Federal circuit courts are split on whether a CBP agent needs "reasonable suspicion" before conducting a forensic search of an electronic device. But Supreme Court precedent clearly states that suspicionless searches are not unconstitutional when public safety is considered. *Skinner v. Ry. Labor Execs.' Ass'n*, 489 U.S. 602 (1989).

A recent CBP directive provides guidance and standard operating procedures regarding forensic searches of electronic devices. CBP 3340-049A, Border Search of Elec. Devices (D.H.S. 2018). The directive states that CBP officers may detain electronic devices, or copies of the information contained within these devices, for a reasonable period time, not to exceed five days. This directive raises the concern that travelers may be required to turn over contact tracing data stored on their phone to CBP officers. Note that the directive has been challenged in federal court and is currently awaiting appeal. *Alasaad v. Nielsen*, 419 F.Supp.3d 142 (D. Mass. 2019).

Searches in Schools

Another exception to the general warrant requirement applies to searches by non-law-enforcement government officials in public schools (i.e., school officials). Within this context, school officials have broad powers to conduct searches as long as those searches are reasonable. Searches by individuals in private schools are not governed by the Fourth Amendment. State regulation of searches in private schools varies. (See US DOE 2009.)

Related Federal Privacy Statutes

Outside the Fourth Amendment context, certain laws provide protections against government collection of and access to personal data. The USA Freedom Act of 2015, for example, bans the government's bulk collection of internet metadata and telephonic records, which was previously allowed under Section 215 of the USA Patriot Act. The government must now identify with specificity the identity of a person, account, address, or personal device when requesting records. The law allows for the acquisition of data by two degrees of separation—or "hops"—from targeted individuals. If a centralized system in contact tracing is used, it is unclear whether the government may need to resort to this provision since it would likely have consent from individuals to collect and use the data.

The Privacy Act of 1974 also regulates the collection, use, and disclosure of personal data, but applies only to federal agencies (and their contractors), not to state or local agencies. 5 U.S.C. § 552a. The Act protects against disclosure of individually identifying "record[s]" that are kept within a "system of records." The Act limits disclosure of information "except pursuant to a written request by, or with prior written consent of, the individual to whom the record pertains." Certain disclosures are exempt from the Act's applicability. Pertinent disclosure exceptions are for records required to be disclosed under the. Freedom of Information Act (FOIA) or disclosures "to a person pursuant to a showing of compelling circumstances affecting the health or safety of an individual." A disclosure under FOIA, however, would not include information in "personnel and medical files and similar files" when disclosure "would constitute a clearly unwarranted invasion of personal privacy." FOIA Guide, 2004 Edition:

Exemption 6. If non-anonymized data are turned over to the federal or state governments, it is important to consider whether PII would be protected from disclosure under FOIA or state freedom of information laws.

Consent

User consent is a cross-cutting issue for evaluating many of the laws and regulations governing personal information privacy discussed in the prior sections. In general, privacy laws can be justified on the grounds that an individual should have the option to control, with various types and degrees of limitation, the collection, use, retention, and/or disclosure of information pertaining to that individual by others. As such, many privacy laws start from the premise that, absent an individual's consent, use or disclosure of that individual's PII is impermissible except for certain enumerated purposes deemed to outweigh the individual's privacy interests.

Consent, like agreements in general, can be manifest in different ways in specific circumstances. In some cases, an affirmative action—such as a signature—is needed to demonstrate consent. In other cases, inaction—such as declining to "unsubscribe" from receiving certain unsolicited emails—constitutes consent. Where a law requires a "written" signature, in all but a few contexts, the signature may be executed electronically. In the United States, that means the "signature" may consist of any of the following: "an electronic sound, symbol, or process," so long as it is "attached to or logically associated with a contract or other record and executed or adopted by a person with the intent to sign the record." Electronic Signatures in Global and National Commerce Act (E-SIGN) (15 U.S.C. 7006).

The scope of a consent depends on what was deemed to be understood by the consenting party. That is least clear when the consent is inferred from inactivity, even if terms stating the consequences of inactivity have been provided. The scope of consent is most clear when the terms agreed to have been presented to or provided by the consenting party in a conspicuous, documented manner and a record exists of those terms. Courts uphold the validity of clickthrough agreements because users are deemed to review the terms to which they respond by clicking "I agree."

But where terms are ambiguous or confusing, buried in other text, or presented obscurely, the "I agree" action may not mean the user actually agreed to specific terms.

Terms of Use and Privacy Policies for apps are often written in complicated or nuanced language, with key points difficult to discern. Moreover, they are generally hard to read on a mobile device. Many users of mobile phone apps agree to such terms without even attempting to read or to understand them. As such, it is often questionable whether an app user has knowingly agreed to all the terms of those documents. Presentation of terms in large typeface, short sentences, simple language, and direct disclosures makes user consent more meaningful.

For contact tracing apps that collect PII and/or PHI, consent will overcome the restrictions of many if not most privacy laws, provided the consent is freely given, reflects a full understanding of the terms for use, collection, and disclosure of the information, and is confirmed by an affirmative act, such as a click that may be executed only upon a complete reading of Terms of Use and Privacy Policies. Whether consent may be deemed "freely given" in certain circumstances depends on contextual understandings of party relationships, including the employer-employee and government-citizen relationships.

Anti-discrimination and Individual Freedom Laws

Any measure taken to protect public health and safety must comply with the Constitution and civil rights laws, such as the ADA, that prohibit discrimination against persons in certain protected categories, such as race, gender, religion, or disability. In addition, certain implementations of DCTT could be challenged under a variety of individual freedom protections.

Anti-discrimination Laws

In general, it would be impermissible to use DCTT in a way that either targets or excludes people on the basis of their membership in one of these protected categories.

When motivated by animus against a protected class as defined by law and not narrowly tailored to advance a compelling government interest, a discriminatory regulation would be considered unconstitutional under the Equal Protection Clause of the Fourteenth Amendment to the US Constitution. See *Jew Ho v. Williamson*, 103 F.10 C.C.N.D. Cal. (1900) (striking down a quarantine imposed by San Francisco in response to an outbreak of bubonic plague because it was racially motivated); see also *Church of Lukumi Babalu Aye v. Hialeah*, 508 U.S. 520 (1993) (supposed public health measure unconstitutional because it targeted the practices of one religion).

The risk of unintentional, yet illegal discrimination in using DCTT is a real possibility. Recent studies of infection rates among the population have revealed a larger-than-proportional infection rate among certain minority communities, such as Latinx, African American, and American Indian communities (NYC DOH 2020). Programs that target specific racial, ethnic, tribal, or religious groups may raise constitutional and other legal concerns.

Religious Freedom Laws

The use of DCTT may also raise concerns about religious freedom. For example, there may be religious objections to restrictions on gathering for worship, carrying a mobile phone, or the use of imaging technology. Under current Supreme Court precedent, generally applicable laws that do not discriminate against religion on their face do not violate the Free Exercise Clause of the First Amendment, even if those laws have an incidental effect on the exercise of religion. *Employment Div. Dept. of Human Resources of Oregon v. Smith*, 494 U.S. 872 (1990). These laws need not be justified by compelling government interest (the "strict scrutiny" standard of review); the government need only show that they are rationally related to a legitimate interest. On the other hand, laws that are not neutral and not of general applicability must be justified by compelling government interest and must be narrowly tailored to advance that interest if it burdens religious practices—a very tough hurdle to overcome. *Church of Lukumi Babalu Aye v. Hialeah*, 508 U.S. 520 (1993).

This general approach, however, is disrupted in some contexts by statutes adopted to provide greater protection to religious freedom. The federal Religious Freedom Restoration Act (RFRA) requires strict scrutiny for federal actions that burden religion, and many states have adopted "state RFRAs" that do the same for actions by state and local governments. The Religious Land Use and Institutionalized Persons Act, which extends similar protections to persons confined to an institution such as a prison, jail, or mental health facility, may also be relevant. 42 U.S.C. § 2000cc.

Under either standard of review, courts will examine whether a government action imposes a substantial burden on religious exercise; if not, no religious freedom violation has occurred. Such a finding is unlikely for DCTT programs absent evidence that the government is using the digital information to take action against religious persons that is not necessary to avoid the spread of a serious disease. Nevertheless, legal challenges on religious freedom grounds cannot be ruled out.

Legislative Recommendations

- Congress should enact new legislation, specifically tailored to facilitate the use of DCTT as part of the public health response to COVID-19, while also protecting user privacy and ensuring data security.

- Congress should require DCTT developers to disclose to users, in clear language, the nature of the information that would be collected, how it would be collected, how it would be stored, and for what purposes it may be used.

- While the rollout of DCTT should initially employ an opt-in authorization approach, the feasibility, acceptability, and value of opt-out approaches should continue to be evaluated. As such, opt-out approaches to consent should not be precluded by legislation.

- Congress should prohibit the commercial use of data collected for COVID-19 response by DCTT.

- Congress should prohibit discrimination on the basis of data collected by DCTT.

- If Congress is unable to enact suitable legislation, state legislatures should work toward enacting similar laws for their jurisdictions. A "model" state law should be rapidly developed to facilitate nationwide uniformity of legal requirements.

FIVE

Recommendations

Public Health

Characteristics That Make Data Useful to
Public Health for Reducing Disease Transmission

- Technologies or apps with the goal of enhancing public health capacity to identify cases and trace contacts in order to control the spread of SARS-CoV-2 should be designed to match functionality with that goal.

- Technologies or apps may produce some false negatives or false positives, but they should be accurate enough that public health authorities feel confident that they support, and don't detract from, contact tracing efforts.

- DCTT approaches for public health should be designed to facilitate the following:

  - Identifying contacts, including those who may not be easily found otherwise.

  - Finding and notifying contacts rapidly, before they develop symptoms if infected.

  - Analyzing the nature of contact to determine whether contact is high, medium, or low risk, to support decisions about whether quarantine should be mandatory, should be voluntary, or is not needed.

  - Following up with cases and contacts so that public health can provide resources to support isolation and quarantine at home.

- Data collected through DCTT should be made available to public health professionals and to researchers in de-identified form to support population-level epidemiologic analysis.

Ethics

Collecting Data to Inform Policy and Practice

- Reviews of DCTT systems must be conducted in part by an independent intermediary that has established the public's trust.

- Those who authorize use of DCTT within a particular jurisdiction or institution should continuously and systematically monitor the technology's performance in that context. This should include monitoring for effectiveness and benefit, monitoring for harms, and monitoring for the fair distribution of both benefits and harms. They should also monitor evidence that is being generated in other contexts about their selected technological solution and about other competing technologies.

- Data should be available to users that would permit them to further investigate their personal risk with public health officials or other health workers to add a layer of protection against unnecessary quarantine.

Public Trust and Public Attitudes

- More research into public attitudes is needed. In particular, in-depth qualitative research should examine public attitudes about perceptions of trust in DCTT among different communities, which features of DCTT influence trust, and the extent to which people are willing to provide different types of data through DCTT to help their community.

- States and localities that are considering adopting DCTT should engage with the public to increase their understanding of the acceptability of DCTT design features and uses among diverse communities.

Designing Flexible Technology to Maximize
Public Health Utility While Respecting Other Values

- Technology companies should not alone control the terms, conditions, or capabilities of DCTT, nor should they presume to know what may be acceptable to members of the public.

- A "values in design" approach to development of DCTT should be adopted (Flanagan, Howe, and Nissenbaum 2008; Knobel and Bowker 2011). Robust public- and user-engagement activities should be pursued to identify and incorporate, to the extent possible, a range of values into the design of the technology. These values may include privacy, but also autonomy, efficiency, equity, or others. Technology design should reflect an appropriate balance and prioritization of identified values.

- Technology design should not be static, but should be capable of evolving depending upon local conditions, new evidence, and changing preferences and priorities.

- DCTT should be designed to have a base set of features that protect privacy, with layers of additional capabilities that users may choose to activate. An initial default should be that user location data are not shared, but users should be provided with easy mechanisms and prompts to allow for opting-in to this capability, with encouragement to the public if and as it is shown to be critical to achieving public health goals.

Policy Positions to Advance Widespread
Use of Digital Contact Tracing Technologies

- DCTT use should not be mandated at this time given uncertainty about potential harms and benefits. Additional technology, user, and real-world testing is needed.

- Incentives can be a useful complement to encouragements; however, any incentives for users to install and use DCTT must be equitable, should not be coercive, and should align with effective use of the technology.

- Trusted leaders should be enlisted to communicate effectively with the public about DCTT and encourage its use, should the technology demonstrate some potential. The limits of knowledge regarding effectiveness should also be explained along with what will be done to improve technological capabilities as understanding evolves.

Disclosure and Authorization/Consent

- A clear and concise module consisting of basic disclosure and voluntary authorization should be developed to accompany DCTT. This module should not take the form of "clickwrap" terms of service or end-user agreements but rather provide only essential information necessary for an individual to make a decision. More detailed disclosures (such as FAQs in plain language) should be made easily accessible to those who wish to learn more, with no hidden surprises.

- An opt-in approach to authorization should be instituted to accompany initial DCTT rollout. The feasibility and value of opt-out approaches should continue to be evaluated, informed by what is technologically possible, what local assessments of benefits and harms of the technology reveal over time, and our evolving understanding of the degree to which an opt-out approach is likely to increase or decrease utilization among different populations. Opt-out approaches should not be precluded.

Promoting Equity and Fairness

- A commitment to equity means a commitment to ensuring that the benefits and burdens of DCTT are distributed fairly. Public engagement is an important tool for assessing impact and to rectify inequities.

- States, localities, and institutions that recommend widespread use of DCTT should provide technology (e.g., mobile phones, Bluetooth devices) and free data packages to those who desire but lack access to these devices.

- If there are lower rates of adoption of DCTT systems in some identifiable communities, public health authorities should identify ways to compensate. For example, directing more non-DCTT resources and efforts toward those communities to meet specific needs that are elsewhere being supported by technology.

- If maps are generated based on DCTT to provide the public with the locations that COV+ individuals have visited, steps must be taken to minimize the stigma and potential financial losses that could result from being identified as a hotspot.

Instituting Transparent Governance and Oversight

- Digital surveillance oversight committees should be established expeditiously, with diverse and qualified membership, to provide ethical and regulatory review prior to and concurrent with widespread use of a DCTT system.

- Understandable and publicly accessible rules must guide the collection, access, control, use, storage, and combination of data by government authorities, public and private institutions, and other parties such as public health researchers.

- Only those data that are necessary and relevant for the public health response to COVID-19 should be collected and used.

- Identifiable data should be kept only for the period of time needed for the public health response to COVID-19.

- Identifiable data collected as part of this response should not be shared with anyone other than the relevant public health authorities without additional specific informed consent of individual users.

- Before a government or institution adopts a digital contact tracing program, they should state the conditions under which the digital contact tracing program will be terminated.

- Future use of DCTT to advance public health or other efforts (e.g., use in seasonal flu surveillance) would require independent justification. DCTT designed for public health use should not be used by law or immigration enforcement.

- The principles offered in this guidance document apply both during and following the COVID-19 pandemic.

Legislative

- Congress should enact new legislation, specifically tailored to facilitate the use of DCTT as part of the public health response to COVID-19, while also protecting user privacy and ensuring data security.
- Congress should require DCTT developers to disclose to users, in clear language, the nature of the information that would be collected, how it would be collected, how it would be stored, and for what purposes it may be used.
- While the rollout of DCTT should initially employ an opt-in authorization approach, the feasibility, acceptability, and value of opt-out approaches should continue to be evaluated. As such, opt-out approaches to consent should not be precluded by legislation.
- Congress should prohibit the commercial use of data collected for COVID-19 response by DCTT.
- Congress should prohibit discrimination on the basis of data collected by DCTT.
- If Congress is unable to enact suitable legislation, state legislatures should work toward enacting similar laws for their jurisdictions. A "model" state law should be rapidly developed to facilitate nationwide uniformity of legal requirements.

Resources

US Government Response

White House

The White House and CDC. 16 April 2020. "Opening Up America Again." The White House and the Centers for Disease Control and Prevention. Available at: https://www.whitehouse.gov/openingamerica/.

Congress

A Bill to Protect the Privacy of Consumers' Personal Health Information, Proximity Data, Device Data, and Geolocation Data during the Coronavirus Public Health Crisis. S.3663, 116th Cong. (2019-2020). Available at: https://www.congress.gov/bill/116th-congress/senate-bill/3663.

A Bill to Protect the Privacy of Health Information during a National Health Emergency. S.3749, 116th Cong. (2019-2020). Available at: https://www.congress.gov/bill/116th-congress/senate-bill/3749.

To Protect the Privacy of Health Information during a National Health Emergency. H.R.6866, 116th Cong. (2019-2020). Available at: https://www.congress.gov/bill/116th-congress/house-bill/6866.

Congressional Research Service

Foster, Michael. 16 April 2020. "COVID-19, Digital Surveillance, and Privacy: Fourth Amendment Considerations." Legal Sidebar LSB10449. Congressional Research Service. https://crsreports.congress.gov/product/pdf/LSB/LSB10449.

Mulligan, Stephen P., and Chris D. Linebaugh. 25 March 2019. "Data Protection Law: An Overview." R45631. Congressional Research Service. https://crsreports.congress.gov/product/pdf/R/R45631.

US Department of Health and Human Services (HHS) /
Centers for Disease Control and Prevention (CDC)

CDC. 6 May 2020. "Interim Guidance for Businesses and Employers."
Coronavirus Disease 2019 (COVID-19). Centers for Disease Control and
Prevention. Available at: https://www.cdc.gov/coronavirus/2019-ncov/
community/guidance-business-response.html.

CDC. 3 May 2020. "Discontinuation of Isolation for Persons with COVID-19
Not in Healthcare Settings." Interim Guidance. Coronavirus Disease 2019
(COVID-19). Centers for Disease Control and Prevention. https://www.cdc
.gov/coronavirus/2019-ncov/hcp/disposition-in-home-patients.html.

CDC. 30 April 2020. "Contact Tracing." Get and Keep America Open: Supporting States, Tribes, Localities, and Territories. Centers for Disease
Control and Prevention. https://www.cdc.gov/coronavirus/2019-ncov/php/
open-america/contact-tracing.html.

CDC. 29 April 2020. "Interim Guidelines for Collecting, Handling, and Testing
Clinical Specimens from Persons for Coronavirus Disease 2019 (COVID-
19)." Coronavirus Disease 2019 (COVID-19). Centers for Disease Control
and Prevention. Available at: https://www.cdc.gov/corona-virus/2019-ncov/
lab/guidelines-clinical-specimens.html

CDC. 29 April 2020. "Contact Tracing: Part of a Multipronged Approach to
Fight the COVID-19 Pandemic." Coronavirus Disease 2019 (COVID-19).
Centers for Disease Control and Prevention. https://www.cdc.gov/
coronavirus/2019-ncov/php/principles-contact-tracing.html.

CDC. 28 April 2020. "Preliminary Criteria for the Evaluation of Digital Contact
Tracing Tools for COVID-19." Coronavirus Disease 2019 (COVID-19).
Centers for Disease Control and Prevention. Available at: https://www.cdc
.gov/coronavirus/2019-ncov/downloads/php/prelim-eval-criteria-digital-
contact-tracing.pdf.

CDC. 20 April 2020. "Digital Contact Tracing Tools for COVID-19." Coronavirus Disease 2019 (COVID-19). Centers for Disease Control and Prevention. Available at: https://www.cdc.gov/coronavirus/2019-ncov/downloads/
digital-contact-tracing.pdf

CDC. 6 April 2020. "Operational Considerations for the Identification of
Healthcare Workers and Inpatients with Suspected COVID-19 in Non-US
Healthcare Settings." Coronavirus Disease 2019 (COVID-19). Centers for
Disease Control and Prevention. Available at: https://www.cdc.gov/coron
virus/2019-ncov/hcp/non-us-settings/guidance-identify-hcw-patients.html.

HHS. 2 April 2020. "Notification of Enforcement Discretion under HIPAA to
Allow Uses and Disclosures of Protected Health Information by Business

Associates for Public Health and Health Oversight Activities in Response to COVID-19." 45 CFR Parts 160 and 164. Available at: https://www.hhs.gov/sites/default/files/notification-enforcement-discretion-hipaa.pdf

HHS. 30 March 2020. Notification of Enforcement Discretion for Telehealth Remote Communications during the COVID-19 Nationwide Public Health Emergency. US Department of Health and Human Services, Office of Civil Rights. Available at: https://www.hhs.gov/hipaa/for-professionals/special-topics/emergency-preparedness/notification-enforcement-discretion-telehealth/index.html

CDC. 24 February 2020. "Legal Authorities for Isolation and Quarantine." Centers for Disease Control and Prevention. Available at: https://www.cdc.gov/quarantine/aboutlawsregulationsquarantineisolation.html.

HHS. 26 November 2019. "Public Health Emergency Declaration." Public Health Emergency. US Department of Health and Human Services, Office of the Assistant Secretary for Preparedness and Response. Available at: https://www.phe.gov/Preparedness/legal/Pages/phedeclaration.aspx

CDC. September 2018. "Public Health Surveillance: Preparing for the Future." Centers for Disease Control and Prevention. Available at: https://www.cdc.gov/surveillance/pdfs/Surveillance-Series-Bookleth.pdf

CDC. 2005. "VI. Plan for Surveillance of Contacts of SARS Case, Supplement B: SARS Surveillance." Centers for Disease Control and Prevention. Available at: https://www.cdc.gov/sars/guidance/b-surveillance/contacts.html.

National Commission for the Protection of Human Subjects of Biomedical and Behavioral Research. 1979. "The Belmont Report: Ethical Principles and Guidelines for the Protection of Human Subjects of Research." US Department of Health and Human Services, Office of Human Research Protections. https://www.hhs.gov/ohrp/regulations-and-policy/belmont-report/read-the-belmont-report/index.html.

US Equal Employment Opportunity Commission (EEOC)

EEOC. 7 May 2020. "What You Should Know About COVID-19 and the ADA, the Rehabilitation Act, and Other EEO Laws." US Equal Employment Opportunity Commission. Available at: https://www.eeoc.gov/wysk/what-you-should-know-about-covid-19-and-ada-rehabilitation-act-and-other-eeo-laws.

EEOC. 21 March 2020. "Pandemic Preparedness in the Workplace and the Americans with Disabilities Act." US Equal Employment Opportunity Commission. Available at: https://www.eeoc.gov/laws/guidance/pandemic-preparedness-workplace-and-americans-disabilities-act.

Federal Trade Commission (FTC)

FTC. 2020. "Privacy & Data Security Update: 2019." Federal Trade Commission. https://www.ftc.gov/system/files/documents/reports/privacy-data-security-update-2019/2019-privacy-data-security-report-508.pdf.

FTC. 2012. "Protecting Consumer Privacy in an Era of Rapid Change." FTC Report. Recommendations for Businesses and Policymakers. Federal Trade Commission. https://www.ftc.gov/sites/default/files/documents/reports/federal-trade-commission-report-protecting-consumer-privacy-era-rapid-change-recommendations/120326privacyreport.pdf.

Occupational Safety and Health Administration (OSHA)

OSHA. April 2020. "Guidance on Preparing Workplaces for COVID-19." OSHA 3990-03 2020. Department of Labor, Occupational Safety and Health Act of 1970. Available at: https://www.osha.gov/Publications/OSHA3990.pdf.

Customs and Border Protection (CBP)

CBP. 4 January 2018. "Border Search of Electronic Media." US Customs and Border Protection CDP DIRECTIVE NO. 3340-049A. Available at: https://www.cbp.gov/sites/default/files/assets/documents/2018-Jan/CBP-Directive-3340-049A-Border-Search-of-Electronic-Media-Compliant.pdf

Other Governmental and Nongovernmental Organizations
Contact Tracing / Surveillance: Plans/Methods

Simmons-Duffin, Selena. 7 May 2020. "States Nearly Doubled Plans for Contact Tracers since NPR Surveyed Them 10 Days Ago." NPR. Available at: https://www.npr.org/sections/health-shots/2020/04/28/846736937/we-asked-all-50-states-about-their-contact-tracing-capacity-heres-what-we-learned.

Resolve to Save Lives. 2020. "COVID-19 Contact Tracing Playbook." Vital Strategies. Available at: https://contacttracingplaybook.resolvetosavelives.org/.

Simpson, Erin, and Adam Conner. 22 April 2020. "Digital Contact Tracing to Contain the Coronavirus." Center for American Progress. Available at: https://www.americanprogress.org/issues/technology-policy/news/2020/04/22/483521/digital-contact-tracing-contain-coronavirus/.

Watson, Crystal, Anita Cicero, James Blumenstock, and Michael Fraser. 10 April 2020. "A National Plan to Enable Comprehensive COVID-19 Case Finding and Contact Tracing in the US." Johns Hopkins Bloomberg School of Public Health: Center for Health Security and the Association of State and Territorial Health Officials. Available at: https://www.centerforhealthsecurity.org/our-work/pubs_archive/pubs-pdfs/2020/200410-national-plan-to-contact-tracing.pdf.

Africa CDC. 9 April 2020. "Guidance on Contact Tracing for COVID-19 Pandemic." Manuals, Guidelines & Frameworks. African Union: Africa CDC. Available at: https://africacdc.org/download/guidance-on-contact-tracing-for-covid-19-pandemic/

PIH. 4 April 2020. "Part I: Testing, Contact Tracing and Community Management of COVID-19." PIH Guide | COVID-19. STOP COVID. Partners in Health. Available at: https://www.pih.org/sites/default/files/2020-04/PIH_Guide_COVID_Part_I_Testing_Tracing_Community_Managment_4_4.pdf.

Hellewell, Joel, Sam Abbott, Amy Gimma, et al. 28 February 2020. "Feasibility of Controlling COVID-19 Outbreaks by Isolation of Cases and Contacts." *The Lancet Global Health* 8: e488–96. Available at: https://doi.org/10.1016/S2214-109X(20)30074-7

Contact Tracing: Ethics/Principles/Guidance

Center for Democracy & Technology (CDT)–https://cdt.org/insights/
CDT. 30 April 2020. "Statement of the Center for Democracy & Technology Regarding Use of Data to Fight COVID-19." Center for Democracy & Technology. https://cdt.org/wp-content/uploads/2020/04/CDT-Statement-Regarding-Use-of-Data-to-Fight-COVID-19.pdf.
Shetty, Ridhi. 23 April 2020. "Data Use in the Fight against COVID-19 Should Treat People Equitably, Not Exacerbate Long-Standing Disparities." Center for Democracy & Technology. https://cdt.org/insights/data-use-in-the-fight-against-covid-19-should-treat-people-equitably-not-exacerbate-long-standing-disparities/.

Greenwood, Dazza, Gregory Nadeau, Pagona Tsormpatzoudi, Bryan Wilson, Jeffrey Saviano, and Alex "Sandy" Pentland. 30 April 2020. "COVID-19 Contact Tracing Privacy Principles." *MIT Computational Law Report.* Available at: https://law.mit.edu/pub/covid19contacttracingprivacy-principles/release/7.

Editorial Board. 29 April 2020. "Show Evidence That Apps for COVID-19 Contact-Tracing Are Secure and Effective." *Nature* 580 (7805): 563–563. https://doi.org/10.1038/d41586-020-01264-1.

"Joint Statement on Contact Tracing." 19 April 2020. Available at: https://cryptobriefing.com/wp-content/uploads/2020/04/Joint-Statement-from-Researchers.pdf

Hinch, Robert, Will Probert, Anel Nurtay, Michelle Kendall, Chris Wymant,

Matthew Hall, Katrina Lythgoe, et al. 16 April 2020. "Effective Configurations of a Digital Contact Tracing App: A Report to NHSX." Available at: https://github.com/BDI-pathogens/covid-19_instant_tracing/blob/master/Report–Effective Configurations of a Digital Contact Tracing App.pdf

Kahn Gilmor, Daniel. 16 April 2020. "Principles for Technology-Assisted Contact-Tracing." White Paper. American Civil Liberties Union. https://www.aclu.org/report/aclu-white-paper-principles-technology-assisted-contact-tracing

Carroll, Anna, and Samantha Stroman. 16 April 2020. "Find My Friends in a Pandemic: The Future of Contact Tracing in America." CSIS Commission on Strengthening America's Health Security. April 16, 2020. https://healthsecurity.csis.org/articles/find-my-friends-in-a-pandemic-the-future-of-contact-tracing-in-america/.

Electronic Privacy Information Center. Testimony to Congress. 15 April 2020. "EPIC to Congress: Establish Privacy Safeguards for Digital Contact Tracing." https://epic.org/testimony/congress/EPIC-HEC-Contact-Tracing-Apr2020.pdf.

Crocker, Andrew, Kurt Opsahl, and Bennett Cyphers. 10 April 2020. "The Challenge of Proximity Apps for COVID-19 Contact Tracing." Electronic Frontier Foundation. April 10, 2020. https://www.eff.org/deeplinks/2020/04/challenge-proximity-apps-covid-19-contact-tracing.

Hart, Vi, Divya Siddarth, Bethan Cantrell, Lila Tretikov, Peter Eckersley, John Langford, Scott Leibrand, et al. 3 April 2020. "Outpacing the Virus: Digital Response to Containing the Spread of COVID-19 While Mitigating Privacy Risks." Whitepaper 5. COVID-19 Rapid Response Impact Initiative. Edmond J. Safra Center for Ethics. https://drive.google.com/file/d/1vIN2AX-DDNW-SoaHq8xsoRJ2jkR_CckX/view.

Raskar, Ramesh, Isabel Schunemann, Rachel Barbar, Kristen Vilcans, Jim Gray, Praneeth Vepakomma, Suraj Kapa, Andrea Nuzzo, Rajiv Gupta et al. 19 March 2020. "Apps Gone Rogue: Maintaining Personal Privacy in an Epidemic." White Paper. Private Kit: MIT. https://arxiv.org/pdf/2003.08567.pdf.

General (not COVID-19 specific) Statements of Principles /
Legal Frameworks / Other Information

Nuffield Council on Bioethics. 2020. "Guide to the Ethics of Surveillance and Quarantine for Novel Coronavirus." https://www.nuffieldbioethics.org/assets/pdfs/Guide-to-the-ethics-of-surveillance-and-quarantine-for-novel-coronavirus.pdf

Schwartz, Adam. 2020. "How EFF Evaluates Government Demands for New Surveillance Powers." Electronic Frontier Foundation. April 3, 2020. https://www.eff.org/deeplinks/2020/04/how-eff-evaluates-government-demands-new-surveillance-powers.

WHO. 2 April 2020. "Coronavirus Disease 2019 (COVID-19)." Situation Report 73. World Health Organization. https://www.who.int/docs/default-source/coronaviruse/situation-reports/20200402-sitrep-73-covid-19.pdf.

Nuffield Council on Bioethics. 17 March 2020. "Ethical Considerations in Responding to the COVID-19 Pandemic." Rapid Policy Briefing. Nuffield Council on Bioethics. https://www.nuffieldbioethics.org/assets/pdfs/Ethical-considerations-in-responding-to-the-COVID-19-pandemic.pdf.

Nuffield Council on Bioethics. 28 January 2020. "Research in Global Health Emergencies: Ethical Issues." https://www.nuffieldbioethics.org/assets/pdfs/RGHE_full_report1.pdf

Vota, Wayan. 4 December 2019. "Every African Country's National eHealth Strategy or Digital Health Policy." ICT Works. https://www.ictworks.org/african-national-ehealth-strategy-policy/

ENISA. 3 December 2019. "Pseudonymisation Techniques and Best Practices." European Union Agency for Cybersecurity. https://www.enisa.europa.eu/publications/pseudonymisation-techniques-and-best-practices

"Mobile Cellular Subscriptions (per 100 People)." 2018. World Telecommunication/ICT Development Report. International Telecommunication Union. https://data.worldbank.org/indicator/IT.CEL.SETS.P2.

Levinson-Waldman, Rachel. 2018. "Cellphones, Law Enforcement, and the Right to Privacy." Brennan Center for Justice, New York University School of Law. https://www.brennancenter.org/sites/default/files/2019-08/Report_Cell_Surveillance_Privacy.pdf

Code of Federal Regulations: Part 46–Protection of Human Subjects (45 CFR 46, US Department of Health and Human Services)

General Data Protection Regulation (REGULATION (EU) 2016/679 (GDPR), European Union)

European Data Protection Supervisor. "Necessity and Proportionality." https://edps.europa.eu/data-protection/our-work/subjects/necessity-proportionality_en

ISO/IEC 38505-1:2017 Information technology—Governance of IT—Governance of data—Part 1: Application of ISO/IEC 38500 to the governance of data (2017, International Organization for Standardization (ISO))

WHO. 2016. "WHO Guidance for Managing Ethical Issues in Infectious Disease Outbreaks." World Health Organization. https://www.who.int/ethics/publications/infectious-disease-outbreaks/en/

CIOMS. 2016. "International Ethical Guidelines for Health-Related Research Involving Humans.–Guideline 22: Use of Data Obtained from the Online Environment and Digital Tools in Health Related Research." Council for International Organizations of Medical Sciences. https://cioms.ch/wp-content/uploads/2017/01/WEB-CIOMS-EthicalGuidelines.pdf

Principles for Digital Development. 2016. "Principles." https://digitalprinciples.org/principles/

GA4GH. 2014. "Framework for Responsible Sharing of Genomic and Health-Related Data." Global Alliance for Genomics & Health. 9 December 2014. https://www.ga4gh.org/genomic-data-toolkit/regulatory-ethics-toolkit/framework-for-responsible-sharing-of-genomic-and-health-related-data/

WHO and PATH. 2013. "Planning an Information Systems Project: A Toolkit for Public Health Managers." World Health Organization & PATH. https://path.azureedge.net/media/documents/TS_opt_ict_toolkit.pdf

ASTHO. 2012. "Public Health Collection, Use, Sharing, and Protection of Information." Issue Brief. ASTHO Legal Preparedness Series. Association of State and Territorial Health Officials. https://www.astho.org/Programs/Preparedness/Public-Health-Emergency-Law/Public-Health-and-Information-Sharing-Toolkit/Collection-Use-Sharing-and-Protection-Issue-Brief/.

Cavoukian, Ann. 2010. "Privacy by Design: The 7 Foundational Principles." Ontario, Canada: Information and Privacy Commissioner of Canada. https://iapp.org/media/pdf/resource_center/pbd_implement_7found_principles.pdf.

PHLS. 2002. "Principles of the Ethical Practice of Public Health." Public Health Leadership Society. https://www.apha.org/-/media/files/pdf/membergroups/ethics/ethics_brochure.ashx.

National Commission for the Protection of Human Subjects of Biomedical and Behavioral Research. 1979. "The Belmont Report: Ethical Principles and Guidelines for the Protection of Human Subjects of Research." US Dept of Health & Human Services, Office of Human Research Protections. https://www.hhs.gov/ohrp/regulations-and-policy/belmont-report/read-the-belmont-report/index.html.

Reopening Proposals/Plans (Broad)

United Kingdom Cabinet Office. 2020. "Our Plan to Rebuild: The UK Government's COVID-19 Recovery Strategy." 12 May 2020. https://www.gov.uk/government/publications/our-plan-to-rebuild-the-uk-governments-covid-19-recovery-strategy/our-plan-to-rebuild-the-uk-governments-covid-19-recovery-strategy#fourteen-supporting-programmes

Shannon, Joel, Lorenzo Reyes, and Doyle Rice. 2020. "Are Lockdowns Being Relaxed in My State? Here's How America Is Reopening amid the Coronavirus Pandemic." *USA TODAY*. May 21, 2020. https://www .usatoday.com/story/news/health/2020/04/19/coronavirus-lockdown-reopening-states-us-texas-florida/5155269002/.

Romer, Paul. 2020. "Roadmap to Responsibly Reopen America." 23 April 2020. https://roadmap.paulromer.net/paulromer-roadmap-report.pdf

Governor Larry Hogan. 24 April 2020. "Maryland Strong: Roadmap to Recovery." https://governor.maryland.gov/wp-content/uploads/2020/04/ MD_Strong.pdf

NGA and ASTHO. 21 April 2020. "Roadmap to Recovery: A Public Health Guide for Governors." National Governors Association and American State and Territorial Health Officials. https://www.nga.org/wp-content/ uploads/2020/04/NGA-Report.pdf

Allen, Danielle, Julius Krein, Ganesh Sitaraman, and E. Glen Weyl. 2020. "National Covid-19 Testing Action Plan." The Rockefeller Foundation. https://www.rockefellerfoundation.org/wp-content/uploads/2020/04/ TheRockefellerFoundation_WhitePaper_Covid19_4_22_2020.pdf.

Edmond J. Safra Center for Ethics, Harvard Univerity–White Papers
Allen, Danielle, Sharon Block, Joshua Cohen et al. 20 April 2020. "Roadmap to Pandemic Resilience." https://ethics.harvard.edu/files/center-for-ethics/files/roadmaptopandemicresilience_updated_4.20.20_0.pdf

Allen, Danielle, Lucas Stanczyk, Rajiv Sethi, Glen Weyl. 25 March 2020. "When Can We Go Out?" https://drive.google.com/ file/d/1gf21eYeNWwrR9OO5nzxn1jlv-RTmHkto/view

Mulheirn, Ian, Sam Alvis, Lizzie Insall, James Browne, Christina Palmou. 20 April 2020. "A Sustainable Exit Strategy: Managing Uncertainty, Minimising Harm." Tony Blair Institute for Global Change. https://institute.global/ sites/default/files/inline-files/A%20Sustainable%20Exit%20Strategy%2C% 20Managing%20Uncertainty%20Minimising%20Harm.pdf

Emanuel, Zeke, Neera Tanden, Adam Conner, Erin Simpson, Nicole Rapfogel, and Maura Calsyn. 2020. "A National and State Plan to End the Coronavirus Crisis." Center for American Progress. April 3, 2020. https:// www.americanprogress.org/issues/healthcare/news/2020/04/03/482613/ national-state-plan-end-coronavirus-crisis/.

Gottlieb, Scott, Caitlin Rivers, Mark McClellan, Lauren Silvis, and Crystal Watson. 2020. "National Coronavirus Response: A Road Map to Reopening." American Enterprise Institute. https://www.aei.org/research-products/ report/national-coronavirus-response-a-road-map-to-reopening/.

Digital Contact Tracing Experiences from Other Countries
Multiple

Woodhams, Samuel. 12 May 2020. "COVID-19 Digital Rights Tracker." Top10VPN. https://www.top10vpn.com/research/investigations/covid-19-digital-rights-tracker/

Fahim, Kareem, Min Joo Kim, and Steve Hendrix. 2 May 2020. "Cellphone Monitoring Is Spreading with the Coronavirus. So Is an Uneasy Tolerance of Surveillance." *Washington Post* (Washington, DC). https://www.washingtonpost.com/world/cellphone-monitoring-is-spreading-with-the-coronavirus-so-is-an-uneasy-tolerance-of-surveillance/2020/05/02/56f14466-7b55-11ea-a311-adb1344719a9_story.html

Ikram, Umar, Christer Mjåset, M.D., Anne-Marie Boxall, Mylaine Breton, Ines Gravey, Holly Krelle, Véronique Raimond, and Reginald D. Williams II. 30 April 2020. "What Can the U.S. Learn from Innovative Strategies Used in Other Countries to Respond to COVID-19?" The Commonwealth Fund. https://www.commonwealthfund.org/blog/2020/what-can-us-learn-innovative-strategies-used-other-countries-respond-covid-19

Jens-Henrik Jeppesen, and Pasquale Esposito. 29 April 2020. "COVID-19: European Data Collection and Contact Tracing Measures." Center for Democracy & Technology. https://cdt.org/insights/covid-19-european-data-collection-and-contact-tracing-measures/

Africa CDC. 9 April 2020. "Guidance on Contact Tracing for COVID-19 Pandemic." Manuals, Guidelines & Frameworks. African Union: Africa CDC. https://africacdc.org/download/guidance-on-contact-tracing-for-covid-19-pandemic/.

Heneghan, Carl, Jon Brassey, and Tom Jefferson. 6 April 2020. "COVID-19: What Proportion Are Asymptomatic?" Centre for Evidence-Based Medicine. https://www.cebm.net/covid-19/covid-19-what-proportion-are-asymptomatic/

Kharpal, Arjun. 30 March 2020. "Use of Surveillance to Fight Coronavirus Raises Concerns about Government Power after Pandemic Ends." *CNBC*. https://www.cnbc.com/2020/03/27/coronavirus-surveillance-used-by-governments-to-fight-pandemic-privacy-concerns.html

Canada

"Commissioner Publishes Framework to Assess Privacy-Impactful Initiatives in Response to COVID19." *Office of the Privacy Commissioner of Canada*. 17 April 2020. https://www.priv.gc.ca/en/opc-news/news-and-announcements/2020/an_200417/

China

Kraemer, Moritz U. G., Chia-Hung Yang, Bernardo Gutierrez, Chieh-Hsi Wu, Brennan Klein, David M. Pigott, Open COVID-19 Data Working Group, Louis du Plessis, Nuno R. Faria, Ruoran Li, William P. Hanage, John S. Brownstein, Maylis Layan, Alessandro Vespignani, Huaiyu Tian, Christopher Dye, Oliver G. Pybus, Samuel V. Scarpino. "The Effect of Human Mobility and Control Measures on the COVID-19 Epidemic in China," *Science* 368(6490): 493-497, DOI: 10.1126/science.abb4218

Bi, Qifang, Yongsheng Wu, Shujiang Mei, Chenfei Ye, Xuan Zou, Zhen Zhang, Xiaojian Liu, Lan Wei, Shaun A Truelove, Tong Zhang, Wei Gao, Cong Cheng, Xiujuan Tang, Xiaoliang Wu, Yu Wu, Binbin Sun, Suli Huang, Yu Sun, Juncen Zhang, Ting Ma, Justin Lessler, and Teijian Feng. "Epidemiology and Transmission of COVID-19 in 391 Cases and 1286 of Their Close Contacts in Shenzhen, China: A Retrospective Cohort Study," *The Lancet*, April 27, 2020, DOI:https://doi.org/10.1016/S1473-3099(20)30287-5

Sun, Kaiyuan, and Cécile Viboud. "Impact of contact tracing on SARS-CoV-2 transmission," *The Lancet*, April 27, 2020, DOI:https://doi.org/10.1016/S1473-3099(20)30357-1

Ferretti, Luca, Chris Wymant, Michelle Kendall, Lele Zhao, Anel Nurtay, Lucie Abeler-Dörner, Michael Parker, David Bonsall, and Christophe Fraser. 2020. "Quantifying SARS-CoV-2 Transmission Suggests Epidemic Control with Digital Contact Tracing." *Science* 368 (6491). https://doi.org/10.1126/science.abb6936.

Gan, Nectar, and David Culver. 2020. "China Is Fighting the Coronavirus with a Digital QR code. Here's How It Works." *CNN Business*. April 16, 2020. https://www.cnn.com/2020/04/15/asia/china-coronavirus-qr-code-intl-hnk/index.html

Mozur, Paul, Raymond Zhong and Aaron Krolik. 2020. "In Coronavirus Fight, China Gives Citizens a Color Code, with Red Flags." *New York Times* (New York, NY). March 1, 2020. https://www.nytimes.com/2020/03/01/business/china-coronavirus-surveillance.html

Germany

Schwartz, Matthew S. 2020. "Germany Backs Away from Compiling Coronavirus Contacts in a Central Database." *NPR*. April 27, 2020. https://www.npr.org/sections/coronavirus-live-updates/2020/04/27/846046185/germany-backs-away-from-compiling-coronavirus-contacts-in-a-central-database?utm_medium=RSS&utm_campaign=news

Busvine, Douglas, and Andreas Rinke. 2020. "Germany Flips to Apple-Google

Approach on Smartphone Contact Tracing." *Reuters*. April 26, 2020. https://www.reuters.com/article/us-health-coronavirus-europe-tech/germany-flips-on-smartphone-contact-tracing-backs-apple-and-google-idUSKCN22807J

Hong Kong

" 'StayHomeSafe' Mobile App User Guide," *The Government of the Hong Kong Special Administrative Region*, May 20, 2020.https://www.coronavirus.gov .hk/eng/stay-home-safe.html

India

Dixit, Pranav. 2020. "India's Contact Tracing App Is All But Mandatory. So This Programmer Hacked It So That He Always Appears Safe." BuzzFeed News. May 12, 2020. https://www.buzzfeednews.com/article/pranavdixit/india-aarogya-setu-hacked.

Greenberg, Andy. 2020. "India's Covid-19 Contact Tracing App Could Leak Patient Locations." *WIRED*. May 6, 2020. https://www.wired.com/story/india-covid-19-contract-tracing-app-patient-location-privacy/

Alderson, Elliot. "Aarogya Setu: The Story of a Failure." *Medium*, May 6, 2020. https://medium.com/@fsoc131y/aarogya-setu-the-story-of-a-failure-3a190a18e34

O'Neill, Patrick Howell. "India Is Forcing People to Use Its COVID App, Unlike Any Other Democracy." *MIT Technology Review*. May 6, 2020. https://www.technologyreview.com/2020/05/07/1001360/india-aarogya-setu-covid-app-mandatory/

Israel

Hendrix, Steve, and Ruth Eglash. 2020. "Israel Is Using Cellphone Surveillance to Warn Citizens: You May Already Be Infected." *Washington Post* (Washington, DC), March 19, 2020. https://www.washingtonpost.com/world/middle_east/israel-is-using-cellphone-surveillance-to-warn-citizens-you-may-already-be-infected/2020/03/19/68267294-69e7-11ea-b199-3a9799c54512_story.html

Singapore

"TraceTogether, Safer Together." A Singapore Government Agency Website, accessed May 21, 2020, https://www.tracetogether.gov.sg/

South Korea

Korean Ministry of Health and Welfare. "Confirmed Patient Movement Path Website." Central Accident Remediation Headquarters, accessed May 21, 2020, http://ncov.mohw.go.kr/bdBoardList_Real.do?brdId=1&brdGubun=12&ncvContSeq=&contSeq=&board_id=&gubun=

Kim, Max S. 2020. "Seoul's Radical Experiment in Digital Contact Tracing." *The New Yorker*. April 17, 2020. https://www.newyorker.com/news/news-desk/seouls-radical-experiment-in-digital-contact-tracing

Watson, Ivan, and Sophie Jeong. 2020. "Coronavirus Mobile Apps Are Surging in Popularity in South Korea." *CNN Business*. February 28, 2020. https://edition.cnn.com/2020/02/28/tech/korea-coronavirus-tracking-apps/index.html

United Kingdom

Hern, Alex, and Kate Proctor. 2020 "UK May Ditch NHS Contact-Tracing App for Apple and Google Model." *The Guardian*. May 7, 2020. https://www.theguardian.com/technology/2020/may/07/uk-may-ditch-nhs-contact-tracing-app-for-apple-and-google-model

Lovejoy, Ben. 2020. "Hands-on with UK's NHS Contact Tracing App as the Test Goes Live." *9-5 Mac Blog*. May 7, 2020. https://9to5mac.com/2020/05/07/nhs-contact-tracing/

"Coronavirus Test, Track and Trace Plan Launched on Isle of Wight." Department of Health and Social Care Press Release. May 4, 2020, https://www.gov.uk/government/news/coronavirus-test-track-and-trace-plan-launched-on-isle-of-wight

Leprince-Ringuet, Daphne. 2020. "Contact-Tracing Apps: Why the NHS Said No to Apple and Google's Plan." *ZDNet*. April 28, 2020. https://www.zdnet.com/article/contact-tracing-apps-why-the-nhs-said-no-to-apple-and-googles-plan/

Specific Digital Products/Apps
COVID-19

Vota, Wayan. 2020. Additional Proposed Coronavirus Solutions. Google Document. https://docs.google.com/spreadsheets/d/15hkhdtGNzx70HkO8Y2MOiY83JsHjqxL4MhMGvlA_J6I/edit#gid=579623365

Apple and Google. n.d. "Privacy-Preserving Contact Tracing." Apple. Accessed May 19, 2020. https://www.apple.com/covid19/contacttracing.

Woodhams, Samuel. 12 May 2020. "COVID-19 Digital Rights Tracker."
Top10VPN. https://www.top10vpn.com/research/investigations/
covid-19-digital-rights-tracker/

Starobinski, David, and Johannes Becker. 30 April 2020. "How Apple and Google Will Let Your Phone Warn You If You've Been Exposed to the Coronavirus." The Conversation. Accessed May 21, 2020. http://theconversation
.com/how-apple-and-google-will-let-your-phone-warn-you-if-youve-been-
exposed-to-the-coronavirus-136597.

Morrison, Sara. 2020. "The Apple-Google Contact Tracing Tool Gets a
Beta Release and a New Risk Level Feature." Vox. April 24, 2020. https://
www.vox.com/recode/2020/4/24/21234420/apple-google-contact-tracing-
exposure-notification-update.

Commonwealth Centre for Digital Health. 9 April 2020. "[Webinar] CWCDH
Digital Response to COVID-19." 50:40. https://www.youtube.com/
watch?v=ZyE_KRWLtC8&feature=youtu.be

Johns Hopkins Medicine. 23 April 2020. "Johns Hopkins Medicine Remote
Monitoring Program for Faculty, Staff and Providers Exposed to COVID-
19." Johns Hopkins Medicine Occupational Health Services. https://www
.hopkinsmedicine.org/hse/covid19_emocha

MIT. n.d. "Private Kit: Safe Paths; Privacy-by-Design Covid19 Solutions Using
GPS+Bluetooth for Citizens and Public Health Officials." Safepaths.
Accessed May 20, 2020. https://safepaths.mit.edu/.

Related Disease Detection Projects

"COVID Control." Google Play, accessed May 21, 2020, https://play.google
.com/store/apps/details?id=jhu.edu.JohnsHopkinsCOVIDControl

"COVID Symptom Tracker," Created by Massachusetts General Hospital, the
Harvard T.H. Chan School of Public Health, King's College London and
Stanford University School of Medicine, accessed May 21, 2020, https://
covid.joinzoe.com/us

"See How Your Community Is Moving around Differently Due to COVID-19."
Google COVID-19 Mobility Reports, accessed May 21, 2020, https://www
.google.com/covid19/mobility/

Drew, David A., Long H. Nguyen, Claire J. Steves, Cristina Menni, Maxim
Freydin, Thomas Varsavsky, Carole H. Sudre, M. Jorge Cardoso, Sebastien
Ourselin, Jonathan Wolf, Tim D. Spector, Andrew T. Chan, and COPE
Consortium. 2020. "Rapid Implementation of Mobile Technology for Real-
Time Epidemiology of COVID-19." Science. 05 May 2020. DOI: 10.1126/
science.abc0473

Tress, Luke. 2020. "Maccabi, Medial EarlySign Develop Algorithm to
    Identify High-Risk COVID-19 Cases." *Times of Israel*. April 22, 2020.
    https://www.timesofisrael.com/maccabi-medial-earlysign-develop-algo
    rithm-to-identify-high-risk-covid-19-cases/
"PCR Diagnostic Testing for SARS-CoV-2." Center for Health Security, Johns
    Hopkins Bloomberg School of Public Health, last modified April 17, 2020.
    https://www.centerforhealthsecurity.org/resources/COVID-19/COVID-19-
    fact-sheets/200130-nCoV-diagnostics-factsheet.pdf
Radin, Jennifer M., Nathan E. Wineinger, Eric J. Topol, and Steven R. Steinhubl.
    2020. "Harnessing Wearable Device Data to Improve State-Level Real-
    Time Surveillance of Influenza-Like Illness in the USA: A Population-Based
    Study." *The Lancet*. January 16, 2020. DOI:https://doi.org/10.1016/
    S2589-7500(19)30222-5

Polling

Hargittai, Eszter, Minh Hao Nguyen, Jaelle Fuchs, Jonathan Gruber, Will
    Marler, Amanda Hunsaker, and Gökçe Karaoglu. 2020. "Covid-19 Study
    on Digital Media and the Coronavirus Pandemic." Internet Use and Society
    Division, Institute of Communication and Media Research, University of
    Zurich. http://webuse.org/covid/.
Navigator Research. 2020. "Public Opinion on Coronavirus: Navigator
    Update." *Navigating Coronavirus* (blog). May 21, 2020. https://
    navigatorresearch.org/navigating-coronavirus/.
Russonello, Giovanni. 2020. "Big Government? For Now, Most Americans Say
    Bring It On." *The New York Times*, May 1, 2020, sec. U.S. https://www
    .nytimes.com/2020/05/01/us/politics/coronavirus-spending-polls.html.
"Washington Post-University of Maryland National Poll." 2020. Washington
    Post. April 21, 2020. https://www.washingtonpost.com/context/
    washington-post-university-of-maryland-national-poll-april-21-26-
    2020/3583b4e9-66be-4ed6-a457-f6630a550ddf/.
Kirzinger, Ashley, Liz Hamel, Cailey Muñana, Audrey Kearney, and Mollyann
    Brodie. 2020. "KFF Health Tracking Poll – Late April 2020: Coronavirus,
    Social Distancing, and Contact Tracing." *Kaiser Family Foundation* (blog).
    April 24, 2020. https://www.kff.org/coronavirus-covid-19/issue-brief/
    kff-health-tracking-poll-late-april-2020/.
NYC DOH. 2020. "Age-Adjusted Rates of Lab Confirmed COVID-19 Non-
    hospitalized Cases, Estimated Non-Fatal Hospitalized Cases, and Persons
    Known to Have Died per 100,000 by Race/Ethnicity Group." New York

City Department of Health. https://www1.nyc.gov/assets/doh/downloads/pdf/imm/covid-19-deaths-race-ethnicity-04242020-1.pdf.

Anderson, Monica, and Brooke Auxier. 2020. "Most Americans Don't Think Cellphone Tracking Will Help Limit COVID-19, Are Divided on Whether It's Acceptable." *Pew Research Center* (blog). April 16, 2020. https://www.pewresearch.org/fact-tank/2020/04/16/most-americans-dont-think-cellphone-tracking-will-help-limit-covid-19-are-divided-on-whether-its-acceptable/.

Daly, Kyle. 2020. "Exclusive: Americans Wary of Giving up Data to Fight Coronavirus." Axios. April 3, 2020. https://www.axios.com/exclusive-americans-wary-of-giving-up-data-to-fight-coronavirus-330fc1d9-8b99-4a51-871b-25ee0e0591f2.html.

Elliott, Douglas J., Ana Kreacic, Lorenzo Milans del Bosch, and Lisa Quest. n.d. "Data-Sharing in the Time of Coronavirus." Oliver Wyman Forum. Accessed May 19, 2020. https://www.oliverwymanforum.com/future-of-data/2020/apr/data-sharing-in-the-time-of-coronavirus.html.

Auxier, Brooke, Lee Rainie, Monica Anderson, Andrew Perrin, Madhu Kumar, and Erica Turner. 2019. "Americans and Privacy: Concerned, Confused and Feeling Lack of Control Over Their Personal Information." *Pew Research Center: Internet, Science & Tech* (blog). November 15, 2019. https://www.pewresearch.org/internet/2019/11/15/americans-and-privacy-concerned-confused-and-feeling-lack-of-control-over-their-personal-information/.

EPIC. 2020. "Public Opinion on Privacy." Electronic Privacy Information Center. January 22, 2020. https://epic.org/privacy/survey/.

Pew Research Center. 2020. "Demographics of Mobile Device Ownership and Adoption in the United States." Internet & Technology. Pew Research Center. https://www.pewresearch.org/internet/fact-sheet/mobile/.

Rodrigues, Rafaela, Alina Husain, Amanda Couture-Carron, Leslye E. Orloff, and Nawal H. Ammar. 2018. "Promoting Access to Justice for Immigrant and Limited English Proficient Crime Victims in an Age of Increased Immigration Enforcement: Initial Report from a 2017 National Survey." Washington, DC: National Immigrant Women's Advocacy Project, American University, Washington College of Law. http://niwaplibrary.wcl.american.edu/wp-content/uploads/Immigrant-Access-to-Justice-National-Report.pdf.

Center for Survey Measurement (CSM). MEMORANDUM FOR Associate Directorate for Research and Methodology (ADRM). 2017. "Respondent Confidentiality Concerns," September 20, 2017. https://www2.census.gov/cac/nac/meetings/2017-11/Memo-Regarding-Respondent-Confidentiality-Concerns.pdf.

Pew Research Center. 2017. "U.S. Muslims Concerned About Their Place in Society, but Continue to Believe in the American Dream." Religion & Public Life. Pew Research Center. https://www.pewforum.org/2017/07/26/findings-from-pew-research-centers-2017-survey-of-us-muslims/.

Popular Press

Dixit, Pranav. 2020. "India's Contact Tracing App Is All But Mandatory. So This Programmer Hacked It So That He Always Appears Safe." BuzzFeed News. May 12, 2020.

Mills Rodrigo, Chris. 2020. "Digital Contact Tracing Is Becoming Available, but Is It Effective?" The Hill. May 7, 2020. https://thehill.com/policy/technology/496498-digital-contact-tracing-is-becoming-available-but-is-it-effective.

Ingram, David. 2020. "Apple, Google Push Makers of Coronavirus Apps Not to Record User Location." May 4 2020. NBC News. Accessed May 19, 2020. https://www.nbcnews.com/tech/tech-news/coronavirus-apps-won-t-be-able-record-users-location-apple-n1199586.

McMinn, Sean. 2020. "Mobile Phone Data Show More Americans Are Leaving Their Homes, Despite Orders." NPR. May 1, 2020. https://www.npr.org/2020/05/01/849161820/mobile-phone-data-show-more-americans-are-leaving-their-homes-despite-orders.

Valentino-DeVries, Jennifer, Natasha Singer, and Aaron Krolik. 2020. "A Scramble for Virus Apps That Do No Harm." The New York Times, April 29, 2020, sec. Business. https://www.nytimes.com/2020/04/29/business/coronavirus-cellphone-apps-contact-tracing.html.

Giglio, Mike. 2020. "Would You Sacrifice Your Privacy to Get Out of Quarantine?" The Atlantic, April 22, 2020. https://www.theatlantic.com/politics/archive/2020/04/coronavirus-pandemic-privacy-civil-liberties-911/609172/

Bradshaw, Tim. 2020. "2 Billion Phones Cannot Use Google and Apple Contact-Tracing Tech | Ars Technica." Ars Technica. April 20, 2020. https://arstechnica.com/tech-policy/2020/04/2-billion-phones-cannot-use-google-and-apple-contract-tracing-tech/.

Reston, Maeve, Kristina Sgueglia, and Cheri Mossburg. 2020. "Governors on East and West Coasts Form Pacts to Decide When to Reopen Economies." CNN Politics. April 13, 2020. https://www.cnn.com/2020/04/13/politics/states-band-together-reopening-plans/index.html.

Cochrane, Emily, Claire Cain Miller, and Jim Tankersley. 2020. "Trump Administration Scales Back Paid Leave in Coronavirus Relief Law." The New York Times, April 2, 2020, sec. U.S. https://www.nytimes.com/2020/04/02/us/politics/coronavirus-paid-leave.html.

Kim, Nemo. 2020. "'More Scary than Coronavirus': South Korea's Health
Alerts Expose Private Lives." The Guardian, March 6, 2020, sec. World
news. https://www.theguardian.com/world/2020/mar/06/more-scary-
than-coronavirus-south-koreas-health-alerts-expose-private-lives

Hickey, Matt. 2014. "Carriers Can Now Install Apps On Android Handsets
Without Customers' Permission." Forbes. December 1, 2014. https://www
.forbes.com/sites/matthickey/2014/12/01/carriers-can-now-install-apps-on-
android-handsets-without-customers-permission/.

Commentaries

Giubilini, Alberto. 2020. "Contact-Tracing Apps and the Future COVID-19
Vaccination Should Be Compulsory. Social, Technological, and Pharmaco-
logical Immunisation." *Practical Ethics* (blog). May 6, 2020. http://blo
g.practicalethics.ox.ac.uk/2020/05/contact-tracing-apps-and-the-future-
covid-19-vaccination-should-be-compulsory-social-technological-and-
pharmacological-immunisation/.

Landau, Susan, Christy Lopez, and Laura Moy. 2020. "The Importance of
Equity in Contact Tracing." *Lawfare* (blog). May 1, 2020. https://www
.lawfareblog.com/importance-equity-contact-tracing.

Schaefer, G. Owen, and Angela Ballantyne. 2020. "Downloading COVID-19
Contact Tracing Apps Is a Moral Obligation." *Journal of Medical Ethics
Blog* (blog). May 4, 2020. https://blogs.bmj.com/medical-ethics/2020/05/04/
downloading-covid-19-contact-tracing-apps-is-a-moral-obligation/.

O'Neill, Patrick Howell. 2020. "Five Things We Need to Do to Make Contact
Tracing Really Work." MIT Technology Review. April 28, 2020. https://
www.technologyreview.com/2020/04/28/1000714/five-things-to-make-
contact-tracing-work-covid-pandemic-apple-google/.

Doffman, Zak. 2020. "COVID-19 Contact Tracing: Why Apple And Google
Can't Make This Work." Forbes. April 27, 2020. https://www.forbes.com/
sites/zakdoffman/2020/04/27/this-is-the-contact-tracing-worry-even-apple-
and-google-cant-resolve/.

All Tech is Human. 2020. *The Ethics of Contact Tracing for COVID-19*.
https://www.youtube.com/watch?v=59mKUAVDhdk&t=626s.

Canca, Cansu. 2020. "Why 'Mandatory Privacy-Preserving Digital Contact
Tracing' Is the Ethical Measure against COVID-19." Medium. May 4,
2020. https://medium.com/@cansucanca/why-mandatory-privacy-preserv-
ing-digital-contact-tracing-is-the-ethical-measure-against-covid-19-a0d-
143b7c3b6

Goodman, Bryce. 2020. "COVID and Contact Tracing: When Social Justice

Demands Mass Surveillance." Medium. April 10, 2020. https://medium.
com/@bwgoodman/covid-and-contact-tracing-when-social-justice-demands-
mass-surveillance-18d419b8cc5.

Gray, Rosie, and Caroline Haskins. 2020. "They Were Opposed To Government Surveillance. Then The Coronavirus Pandemic Began." BuzzFeed
News. March 30, 2020. https://www.buzzfeednews.com/article/rosiegray/
they-were-opposed-to-government-surveillance-then-the.

Cegłowski, Maciej. 2020. "We Need A Massive Surveillance Program." *Idle
Words* (blog). March 23, 2020. https://idlewords.com/2020/03/we_need_
a_massive_surveillance_program.htm.

Academic Literature

COVID-19 Specific

Abeler J, Bäcker M, Buermeyer U, Zillessen H (2020). COVID-19 Contact
Tracing and Data Protection Can Go Together. JMIR mHealth and
uHealth 8(4): e19359. doi: 10.2196/19359.

Altmann S, Milsom L, Zillessen H et al (2020). Acceptability of App-Based
Contact Tracing for COVID-19: Cross-Country Survey Evidence. Preprint.

Berke A, Bakker M, Vepakomma P, Larson K, Pentland A (2020). Assessing
Disease Exposure Risk with Location Data: A Proposal for Cryptographic
Preservation of Privacy. arXiv, arXiv:2003.14412–March 2020.

Bonsail D, Parker M, Fraser C (2020). Sustainable Containment of COVID-19
Using Smartphones in China: Scientific and Ethical Underpinnings for
Implementation of Similar Approaches in Other Settings. Unpublished
working paper.

Bradshaw WJ, Alley EC, Huggins JH, Lloyd AL, Esvelt KM (2020). Bidirectional
Contact Tracing Is Required for Reliable COVID-19 Control. Preprint via
MedRxiv.

Braithwaite I, Callender T, Bullock M, Aldridge R (2020). Automated and
Semi-Automated Contact Tracing: Protocol for a Rapid Review of Avail-
able Evidence and Current Challenges to Inform the Control of COVID-19.
Preprint via medRxiv. doi: https://doi.org/10.1101/2020.04.14.20063636.

Bulchandani Bannerjee V, Shivam S, Moudgalya S, Sondhi SL (2020). Digital
Herd Immunity and COVID-19. Preprint via medRxiv. doi: https://doi.org/
10.1101/2020.04.15.20066720.

Cheng H, Jian S, Liu D (2020). Contact Tracing Assessment of COVID 19
Transmission Dynamics in Taiwan and Risk at Different Exposure Periods
Before and After Symptom Onset. JAMA Internal Medicine. doi:10.1001/
jamainternmed.2020.2020.

Cho H, Ippolito D, Yu YW (2020). Contact Tracing Mobile Apps for COVID-19: Privacy Considerations and Related Trade-offs. https://arxiv.org/pdf/2003.11511.pdf.

Devakumar D, Geordan S, Bhopal SS, Abubakar I (2020). Racism and discrimination in COVID-19 responses. The Lancet 395(10231): 1194. doi: 10.1016/S0140-6736(20)30792-3.

Drew D, Nguyen L, Steves C et al. (2020). Rapid Implementation of Mobile Technology for Real-Time Epidemiology of COVID-19. Science, published online May 5, 2020.

Ferretti L, Wymant C, Kendall M et al. (2020) Quantifying SARS-CoV-2 Transmission Suggests Epidemic Control with Digital Contact Tracing. Science. doi: 10.1126/science.abb6936.

Fraser C, Abeler-Dörner, L, Ferretti L et al. (2020). Digital Contact Tracing: Comparing the Capabilities of Centralised and Decentralised Data Architectures to Effectively Suppress the COVID-19 Epidemic While Maximizing Freedom of Movement and Maintaining Privacy. Preprint.

Leith DJ, Farrell S (2020). Coronavirus Contact Tracing: Evaluating The Potential Of Using Bluetooth Received Signal Strength For Proximity Detection. Preprint.

Jayant Limaye R, Sauer M, Ali J et al. (2020). Building Trust While Influencing Online COVID-19 Content iIn the Social Media World. The Lancet Digital Health.

Mahmood S, Hasan K, Colder Carras M, Labrique A (2020). Global Preparedness Aagainst COVID-19: We Must Leverage the Power of Digital Health. JMIR Public Health Surveill 2020;6(2):e18980, DOI: 10.2196/18980.

Mello M, Wang CJ (2020) Ethics and Governance for Digital Disease Surveillance. Science. 11 May 2020: eabb9045 DOI: 10.1126/science.abb9045.

Park S, Jeehyun Choi G; Ko H (2020). Information Technology–Based Tracing Strategy in Response to COVID-19 in South Korea—Privacy Controversies. JAMA. doi:10.1001/jama.2020.6602.

Parker M, Fraser C, Abeler-Dörner L, Bonsall D (2020). Ethics of Instantaneous Contract Tracing Using Mobile Phone Apps in the Control of the COVID-19 Pandemic. Journal of Medical Ethics. Published Online, May 4, 2020.

Ethics and Digital Disease Detection

Aiello A, Renson A, Civich P (2020). Social Media– and Internet-Based Disease Surveillance for Public Health. Annual Review of Public Health 41: 101–118. doi: 10.1146/annurev-publhealth-040119-094402.

Ali J, DiStefano M, Coates McCall I, et al. (2019). Ethics of Mobile Phone Surveys to Monitor Non-Communicable Disease Risk Factors in Low- and Middle-Income Countries: A Global Stakeholder Survey. Global Public Health 14(8): 1167–1181.

Ali J, Labrique A, Gionfriddo K et al. (2017) Ethics Considerations in Global Mobile Phone-Based Surveys of Noncommunicable Diseases: A Conceptual Exploration. Journal of Medical Internet Research 19(5): e110. doi: 10.2196/jmir.7326.

Brownstein J, Freifeld C, Madoff L (2009). Digital Disease Detection–Harnessing the Web for Public Health Surveillance. New England Journal of Medicine 360(21): 2153–2157. doi: 10.1056/NEJMp0900702.

Danquah LO, Hasham N, MacFarlane M et al. (2019). Use of a Mobile Application for Ebola Contact Tracing and Monitoring in Northern Sierra Leone: A Proof-of-Concept Study. BMC Infectious Diseases 19: 810.

Degeling C, Carter S, van Oijen A et al. (2020). Community Perspectives on the Benefits and Risks of Technologically Enhanced Communicable Disease Surveillance Systems: A Report on Four Community Juries. BMC Medical Ethics 21, 31. doi: 10.1186/s12910-020-00474-6.

DeJong B, Badou G, Luten J et al. (2019). Ethical Considerations for Movement Mapping to Identify Disease Transmission Hotspots. Emerging Infectious Diseases 25(7): e181421. doi: 10.3201/eid2507.181421.

Denecke K (2017). An Ethical Assessment Model for Digital Disease Detection Technologies. Life Sciences, Society and Policy 13, 16. doi: 10.1186/s40504-017-0062-x.

Genevieve LD, Martani A, Wangmo T et al. (2019). Participatory Disease Surveillance Systems: Ethical Framework. Journal of Medical Internet Research 21(5): e12273. doi:10.2196/12273.

Gilbert G, Degeling C, Johnson J (2017). Communicable Disease Surveillance Ethics in the Age of Big Data and New Technology. Asian Bioethics Review 11: 173-187. doi: 10.1007/s41649-019-00087-1.

Iwaya LH, Li J, Fischer-Hubner S et al. (2019). E-Consent for Data Privacy: Consent Management for Mobile Health Technologies in Public Health Surveys and Disease Surveillance. Studies in health technology and informatics 264: 1223-1227. doi: 10.3233/SHTI190421.

Kostkova P (2018). Disease Surveillance Data Sharing for Public Health: The Next Ethical Frontiers. Life Sciences, Society and Policy 14: 16. doi: 10.1186/s40504-018-0078-x.

Mahmood S, Hasan K, Colder Carras M, Labrique A (2020). Global Preparedness against COVID-19: We Must Leverage the Power of Digital Health. JMIR Public Health Surveillance 6(2):e18980.

Smolinski MS, Crawley AW, Baltrusaitis K et al. (2015). Flu Near You: Crowd-sourced Symptom Reporting Spanning 2 Influenza Seasons. AJPH 105(10): 2124–2130.

Wojcik O, Brownstein J, Chunara R, Johansson M (2014). Public Health for the People: Participatory Infectious Disease Surveillance in the Digital Age. Emerging Themes in Epidemiology 11, 7. doi: 10.1186/1742-7622-11-7.

Other Works

Bernstein J, Holroyd TA, Atwell JE, et al. (2019). Rockland County's Proposed Ban against Unvaccinated Minors: Balancing Disease Control, Trust, and Liberty. Vaccine 37(30): 3933–3935.

Berry SM, Petzold EA, Dull P et al. (2017). A Response Adaptive Randomization Platform Trial for Efficient Evaluation of Ebola Virus Treatments: A Model for Pandemic Response. Clinical Trials 13(1): 22–30. doi: 10.1177/1740774515621721.

Beukenhorst AL, Schultz DM, McBeth J (2017). Using Smartphones for Research outside Clinical Settings: How Operating Systems, App Developers, and Users Determine Geolocation Data Quality in mHealth Studies. MEDINFO 2017: Precision Healthcare through Informatics.

Bourne P (2015). Confronting the Ethical Challenges of Big Data in Public Health. Plos Computational Biology 11(2): e1004073. doi: 10.1371/journal.pcbi.1004073.

Doerr M, Suver C, Wilbanks J (2016). Developing a Transparent, Participant-Navigated Electronic Informed Consent for Mobile-Mediated Research. (April 22, 2016). Available at SSRN: https://ssrn.com/abstract=2769129 or http://dx.doi.org/10.2139/ssrn.2769129.

Dredze M, Paul MJ, Bergsma S, Tran H (2013). Carmen: A Twitter Geolocation System with Applications to Public Health. Expanding the Boundaries of Health Informatics Using Artificial Intelligence: Papers from the AAAI 2013 Workshop.

Eckhoff PA, Tatem AJ (2015). Digital methods in epidemiology can transform disease control.International Health, Volume 7, Issue 2, March 2015, Pages 77–78, https://doi.org/10.1093/inthealth/ihv013.

Edelstein M, Lee L, Herten-Crabb A, Heymann D, Harper D (2018). Strengthening Global Public Health Surveillance through Data and Benefit Sharing. Emerging Infectious Diseases 24(7): 1324–1330. doi: 10.3201/eid2407.151830.

Faden R, Beauchamp T (1986). A History and Theory of Informed Consent. Oxford University Press. ISBN: 9780199748655.

Fairchild A, Bayer R (2004). Ethics and the Conduct of Public Health Surveillance. Science 303(5658): 631–632.

Flanagan M, Howe DC, Nissenbaum H (2008). Embodying Values in Technology: Theory and Practice. In: Information Technology and Moral Philosophy. van den Hoven J & Weckert J. (eds.) Cambridge, Cambridge University Press. 322–353.

Fraccaro P, Beukenhorst A, Sperrin M et al. (2019). Digital Biomarkers from Geolocation Data in Bipolar Disorder and Schizophrenia: A Systematic Review. Journal of the American Medical Informatics Association, Volume 26, Issue 11, November 2019, Pages 1412–1420.

Furlanello C, Merler S, Menegon S et al. (2002). New WEBGIS Technologies for Geo-location of Epidemiological Data: An Application for the Surveillance of the Risk of Lyme borreliosis Disease. In: Giornale Italiano di Aritmologia e Cardiostimolazione, Special Issue Proceedings of the 15th Int. Congress "The New Frontiers of Arrhythmias," v. 5, n.1, Mar 2002, 241–245.

Gibson DG, Wosu AC, Pariyo GW et al. (2019). Effect of Airtime Incentives on Response and Cooperation Rates in Non-communicable Disease Interactive Voice Response Surveys: Randomised Controlled Trials in Bangladesh and Uganda. BMJ Global Health 4(5).

Knobel C, Bowker GC (2011). Computing Ethics: Values in Design. Communications of the acm. 54(7): 26–28.

Lee R, Cui RR, Muessig KE et al. (2015). Incentivizing HIV/STI Testing: A Systematic Review of the Literature. AIDS and Behavior 18(5): 905–912. doi: 10.1007/s10461-013-0588-8.

Lorchan LT, Wyatt J (2014). mHealth and Mobile Medical Apps: A Framework to Assess Risk and Promote Safer Use. Journal of Medical Internet Research 16(9): e210. doi: 10.2196/jmir.3133.

Mathews S, McShea M, Hanley C et al. (2019). Digital Health: A Path to Validation. Digital Medicine 2:38. doi: 10.1038/s41746-019-0111-3.

Moore S, Tasse A, Thorogood A, et al. (2017). Consent Processes for Mobile App Mediated Research: Systematic Review. JMIR mHealth & uHealth 5(8): e126. DOI: 10.2196/mhealth.7014.

Pallman P, Bedding AW, Choodari-Oskooei B et al. (2018). Adaptive Designs in Clinical Trials: Why Use Them, and How to Run and Report Them. BMC Medicine 16(29).

Rennie S, Buchbinder M, Juengst E et al. (2020). Scraping the Web for Public Health Gains: Ethical Considerations from a 'Big Data' Research Project on HIV and Incarceration. Public Health Ethics. doi: 10.1093/phe/phaa006.

Rithalia A, McDaid C, Suekarran S (2009). Impact of Presumed Consent for Organ Donation on Donation Rates: A Systematic Review. BMJ 2009; 338.

Singer E, Ye C (2012). The Use and Effects of Incentives in Surveys. The ANNALS of the American Academy of Political and Social Science 645(1): 112–141.

Vayena E, Blassime A (2018). Health Research with Big Data: Time for Systemic Oversight. J Law Med Ethics. 2018 Mar; 46(1): 119–129.

Vayena E, Mastroianni A, Kahn J (2012). Ethical Issues in Health Research with Novel Online Sources. American Journal of Public Health 102(12): 2225–2230. doi: 10.2105/AJPH.2012.300813.

Vayena E, Salathé M, Madoff L, Brownstein J (2015). Ethical Challenges of Big Data in Public Health. Plos Computational Biology 11(2): e1003904. doi: 10.1371/journal.pcbi.1003904.

Xafis V, Schaefer GO, Labude MK et al. (2019). An Ethics Framework for Big Data in Health and Research. Asian Bioethics Review volume 11, pages 227–254(2019).

Works Cited

Africa CDC. 2020. "Guidance on Contact Tracing for COVID-19 Pandemic."
Manuals, Guidelines & Frameworks. African Union: Africa CDC. https://
africacdc.org/download/guidance-on-contact-tracing-for-covid-19-
pandemic/.

Aiello, Allison E., Audrey Renson, and Paul N. Zivich. 2020. "Social
Media– and Internet-Based Disease Surveillance for Public Health."
Annual Review of Public Health 41 (1): 101–18. https://doi.org/10.1146/
annurev-publhealth-040119-094402.

Ali, Joseph, Michael J. DiStefano, Iris Coates McCall, Dustin G. Gibson,
Gulam Muhammed Al Kibria, George W. Pariyo, Alain B. Labrique,
and Adnan A. Hyder. 2019. "Ethics of Mobile Phone Surveys to Monitor
Non-Communicable Disease Risk Factors in Low- and Middle-Income
Countries: A Global Stakeholder Survey." Global Public Health 14 (8):
1167–81. https://doi.org/10.1080/17441692.2019.1566482.

Ali, Joseph, Alain B. Labrique, Kara Gionfriddo, George Pariyo, Dustin G.
Gibson, Bridget Pratt, Molly Deutsch-Feldman, and Adnan A. Hyder.
2017. "Ethics Considerations in Global Mobile Phone-Based Surveys of
Noncommunicable Diseases: A Conceptual Exploration." Journal of Medical Internet Research 19 (5): e110. https://doi.org/10.2196/jmir.7326.

Allen, Danielle, Julius Krein, Ganesh Sitaraman, and E. Glen Weyl. 2020.
"National Covid-19 Testing Action Plan." The Rockefeller Foundation.
https://www.rockefellerfoundation.org/wp-content/uploads/2020/04/
TheRockefellerFoundation_WhitePaper_Covid19_4_22_2020.pdf.

Altmann, Samuel, Luke Milsom, Hannah Zillessen, Raffaele Blasone, Frederic
Gerdon, Ruben Bach, Frauke Kreuter, Daniele Nosenzo, Severine Tous-
saert, and Johannes Abeler. 2020. "Acceptability of App-Based Contact
Tracing for COVID-19: Cross-Country Survey Evidence." MedRxiv, May,
2020.05.05.20091587. https://doi.org/10.1101/2020.05.05.20091587.

Anderson, Monica, and Brooke Auxier. 2020. "Most Americans Don't Think
Cellphone Tracking Will Help Limit COVID-19, Are Divided on Whether

It's Acceptable." Pew Research Center (blog). April 16, 2020. https://
www.pewresearch.org/fact-tank/2020/04/16/most-americans-dont-think-
cellphone-tracking-will-help-limit-covid-19-are-divided-on-whether-its-
acceptable/.

Anderson, Monica, and Andrew Perrin. 2017. "Disabled Americans Less
Likely to Use Technology." Pew Research Center (blog). April 7, 2017.
https://www.pewresearch.org/fact-tank/2017/04/07/disabled-americans-
are-less-likely-to-use-technology/.

Apple and Google. n.d. "Privacy-Preserving Contact Tracing." Apple.
Accessed May 19, 2020. https://www.apple.com/covid19/contacttracing.

ASTHO. 2012. "Public Health Collection, Use, Sharing, and Protection of
Information." Issue Brief. ASTHO Legal Preparedness Series. Association
of State and Territorial Health Officials. https://www.astho.org/Programs/
Preparedness/Public-Health-Emergency-Law/Public-Health-and-
Information-Sharing-Toolkit/Collection-Use-Sharing-and-Protection-
Issue-Brief/.

Auxier, Brooke, Lee Rainie, Monica Anderson, Andrew Perrin, Madhu
Kumar, and Erica Turner. 2019. "Americans and Privacy: Concerned,
Confused and Feeling Lack of Control Over Their Personal Information."
Pew Research Center: Internet, Science & Tech (blog). November 15, 2019.
https://www.pewresearch.org/internet/2019/11/15/americans-and-privacy-
concerned-confused-and-feeling-lack-of-control-over-their-personal-infor
mation/.

Barth, Susanne, and Menno D. T. de Jong. 2017. "The Privacy Paradox – Investigating Discrepancies between Expressed Privacy Concerns and Actual
Online Behavior – A Systematic Literature Review." Telematics and Informatics 34 (7): 1038–58. https://doi.org/10.1016/j.tele.2017.04.013.

Bernstein, Justin, Taylor A. Holroyd, Jessica E. Atwell, Joseph Ali, and Rupali
J. Limaye. 2019. "Rockland County's Proposed Ban against Unvaccinated
Minors: Balancing Disease Control, Trust, and Liberty." Vaccine, June.
https://doi.org/10.1016/j.vaccine.2019.05.093.

Berry, Scott M., Elizabeth A. Petzold, Peter Dull, Nathan M. Thielman,
Coleen K. Cunningham, G. Ralph Corey, Micah T. McClain, et al. 2016.
"A Response Adaptive Randomization Platform Trial for Efficient Evalua-
tion of Ebola Virus Treatments: A Model for Pandemic Response." Clinical
Trials (London, England) 13 (1): 22–30. https://doi.org/10.1177/
1740774515621721.

Beukenhorst, A.L., D.M. Schultz, J. McBeth, R. Lakshminarayana, J.C. Sergeant,
and W.G. Dixon. 2017. "Using Smartphones for Research Outside Clinical

Settings: How Operating Systems, App Evelopers, and Users Determine Geolocation Data Quality in MHealth Studies." In MEDINFO 2017: Precision Healthcare through Infomatics, 10–14. IOS Press. http://ebooks .iospress.nl/volumearticle/48095.

Bradshaw, Tim. 2020. "2 Billion Phones Cannot Use Google and Apple Contact-Tracing Tech | Ars Technica." Ars Technica. April 20, 2020. https:// arstechnica.com/tech-policy/2020/04/2-billion-phones-cannot-use-google-and-apple-contract-tracing-tech/.

Canca, Cansu. 2020. "Why 'Mandatory Privacy-Preserving Digital Contact Tracing' Is the Ethical Measure against COVID-19." Medium. May 4, 2020. https://medium.com/@cansucanca/why-mandatory-privacy-preserving-digital-contact-tracing-is-the-ethical-measure-against-covid-19-a0d143b7c3b6.

Cavalier, Robert J., ed. 2011. Approaching Deliberative Democracy: Theory and Practice. Carnegie Mellon University Press.

Cavoukian, Ann. 2010. "Privacy by Design: The 7 Foundational Principles." Ontario, Canada: Information and Privacy Commissioner of Canada. https://iapp.org/media/pdf/resource_center/pbd_implement_7found_principles.pdf.

CDC. 2005. "VI. Plan for Surveillance of Contacts of SARS Case, Supplement B: SARS Surveillance." Centers for Disease Control and Prevention. https:// www.cdc.gov/sars/guidance/b-surveillance/contacts.html.

———. 2020a. "Contact Tracing." Get and Keep America Open: Supporting States, Tribes, Localities, and Territories. Centers for Disease Control and Prevention. https://www.cdc.gov/coronavirus/2019-ncov/php/open-america/contact-tracing.html.

———. 2020b. "Contact Tracing: Part of a Multipronged Approach to Fight the COVID-19 Pandemic." Coronavirus Disease 2019 (COVID-19). Centers for Disease Control and Prevention. https://www.cdc.gov/coronavirus/2019-ncov/php/principles-contact-tracing.html.

———. 2020c. "Interim Guidance for Businesses and Employers." Coronavirus Disease 2019 (COVID-19). Centers for Disease Control and Prevention. https://www.cdc.gov/coronavirus/2019-ncov/community/guidance-business-response.html.

———. 2020d. "Operational Considerations for the Identification of Healthcare Workers and Inpatients with Suspected COVID-19 in Non-US Healthcare Settings." Coronavirus Disease 2019 (COVID-19). Centers for Disease Control and Prevention. https://www.cdc.gov/coronavirus/2019-ncov/hcp/non-us-settings/guidance-identify-hcw-patients.html.

———. 2020e. "Preliminary Criteria for the Evaluation of Digital Contact Tracing Tools for COVID-19." Coronavirus Disease 2019 (COVID-19). Centers for Disease Control and Prevention. https://www.cdc.gov/coronavirus/2019-ncov/downloads/php/prelim-eval-criteria-digital-contact-tracing.pdf.

———. 2020f. "Legal Authorities for Isolation and Quarantine." Centers for Disease Control and Prevention. https://www.cdc.gov/quarantine/aboutlawsregulationsquarantineisolation.html.

———. 2020g. "Discontinuation of Isolation for Persons with COVID-19 Not in Healthcare Settings." Interim Guidance. Coronavirus Disease 2019 (COVID-19). Centers for Disease Control and Prevention. https://www.cdc.gov/coronavirus/2019-ncov/hcp/disposition-in-home-patients.html.

———. 2020h. "COVID-19 Provisional Counts–Weekly Updates by Select Demographic and Geographic Characteristics." CDC National Vital Statistics System. https://www.cdc.gov/nchs/nvss/vsrr/covid_weekly/index.htm.

Center for Survey Measurement (CSM). MEMORANDUM FOR Associate Directorate for Research and Methodology (ADRM). 2017. "Respondent Confidentiality Concerns," September 20, 2017. https://www2.census.gov/cac/nac/meetings/2017-11/Memo-Regarding-Respondent-Confidentiality-Concerns.pdf.

Cheng, Hao-Yuan, Shu-Wan Jian, Ding-Ping Liu, Ta-Chou Ng, Wan-Ting Huang, and Hsien-Ho Lin. 2020. "Contact Tracing Assessment of COVID-19 Transmission Dynamics in Taiwan and Risk at Different Exposure Periods Before and After Symptom Onset." JAMA Internal Medicine, May. https://doi.org/10.1001/jamainternmed.2020.2020.

Cochrane, Emily, Claire Cain Miller, and Jim Tankersley. 2020. "Trump Administration Scales Back Paid Leave in Coronavirus Relief Law." The New York Times, April 2, 2020, sec. U.S. https://www.nytimes.com/2020/04/02/us/politics/coronavirus-paid-leave.html.

Crocker, Andrew, Kurt Opsahl, and Bennett Cyphers. 2020. "The Challenge of Proximity Apps For COVID-19 Contact Tracing." Electronic Frontier Foundation. April 10, 2020. https://www.eff.org/deeplinks/2020/04/challenge-proximity-apps-covid-19-contact-tracing.

Danquah, Lisa O., Nadia Hasham, Matthew MacFarlane, Fatu E. Conteh, Fatoma Momoh, Andrew A. Tedesco, Amara Jambai, David A. Ross, and Helen A. Weiss. 2019. "Use of a Mobile Application for Ebola Contact Tracing and Monitoring in Northern Sierra Leone: A Proof-of-Concept Study." BMC Infectious Diseases 19 (1): 810. https://doi.org/10.1186/s12879-019-4354-z.

de Jong, Bouke C., Badou M. Gaye, Jeroen Luyten, Bart van Buitenen, Emmanuel André, Conor J. Meehan, Cian O'Siochain, et al. 2019. "Ethical Considerations for Movement Mapping to Identify Disease Transmission Hotspots." Emerging Infectious Diseases 25 (7). https://doi.org/10.3201/eid2507.181421.

Devakumar, Delan, Geordan Shannon, Sunil S Bhopal, and Ibrahim Abubakar. 2020. "Racism and Discrimination in COVID-19 Responses." Lancet (London, England) 395 (10231): 1194. https://doi.org/10.1016/S0140-6736(20)30792-3.

Dixit, Pranav. 2020. "India's Contact Tracing App Is All But Mandatory. So This Programmer Hacked It So That He Always Appears Safe." BuzzFeed News. May 12, 2020. https://www.buzzfeednews.com/article/pranavdixit/india-aarogya-setu-hacked.

Doerr, Megan, Christine Suver, and John Wilbanks. 2016. "Developing a Transparent, Participant-Navigated Electronic Informed Consent for Mobile-Mediated Research." SSRN Scholarly Paper ID 2769129. Rochester, NY: Social Science Research Network. https://doi.org/10.2139/ssrn.2769129.

Dredze, Mark, Michael J. Paul, Shane Bergsma, and Hieu Tran. 2013. "Carmen: A Twitter Geolocation System with Applications to Public Health." AAAI Workshops; Workshops at the Twenty-Seventh AAAI Conference on Artificial Intelligence. https://www.aaai.org/ocs/index.php/WS/AAAIW13/paper/view/7085/6497.

Eckhoff, Philip A., and Andrew J. Tatem. 2015. "Digital Methods in Epidemiology Can Transform Disease Control." International Health 7 (2): 77–78. https://doi.org/10.1093/inthealth/ihv013.

EEOC. 2020. "What You Should Know About COVID-19 and the ADA, the Rehabilitation Act, and Other EEO Laws." U.S. Equal Employment Opportunity Commission. May 7, 2020. https://www.eeoc.gov/wysk/what-you-should-know-about-covid-19-and-ada-rehabilitation-act-and-other-eeo-laws.

Electronic Privacy Information Center. Testimony to Congress. 2020. "EPIC to Congress: Establish Privacy Safeguards for Digital Contact Tracing," April 15, 2020. https://epic.org/testimony/congress/EPIC-HEC-Contact-Tracing-Apr2020.pdf.

Elliott, Douglas J., Ana Kreacic, Lorenzo Milans del Bosch, and Lisa Quest. 2020. "Data-Sharing in the Time of Coronavirus." Oliver Wyman Forum. Accessed May 19, 2020. https://www.oliverwymanforum.com/future-of-data/2020/apr/data-sharing-in-the-time-of-coronavirus.html.

Faden, Ruth R., and Tom L. Beauchamp. 1986. A History and Theory of Informed Consent. Oxford University Press.

FCC and FTC. 2017. "FCC-FTC Consumer Protection Memorandum of Understanding." Federal Communications Commission and Federal Trade Commission. https://www.ftc.gov/system/files/documents/cooperation_ agreements/151116ftcfcc-mou.pdf.

Ferretti, Luca, Chris Wymant, Michelle Kendall, Lele Zhao, Anel Nurtay, Lucie Abeler-Dörner, Michael Parker, David Bonsall, and Christophe Fraser. 2020. "Quantifying SARS-CoV-2 Transmission Suggests Epidemic Control with Digital Contact Tracing." Science 368 (6491). https://doi.org/10.1126/ science.abb6936.

Fishkin, James S., and Peter Laslett, eds. 2003. Debating Deliberative Democracy. Blackwell Publisher, Ltd. https://onlinelibrary.wiley.com/doi/book/ 10.1002/9780470690734.

Flanagan, Mary, Daniel C. Howe, and Helen Nissenbaum. 2008. "Embodying Values in Technology: Theory and Practice." In Information Technology and Moral Philosophy, edited by Jeroen van den Hoven and John Weckert, 322–53. Cambridge University Press.

Fraccaro, Paolo, Anna Beukenhorst, Matthew Sperrin, Simon Harper, Jasper Palmier-Claus, Shôn Lewis, Sabine N. Van der Veer, and Niels Peek. 2019. "Digital Biomarkers from Geolocation Data in Bipolar Disorder and Schizophrenia: A Systematic Review." Journal of the American Medical Informatics Association 26 (11): 1412–20. https://doi.org/10.1093/jamia/ ocz043.

Fraser, Christophe, Lucie Abeler-Dörner, Luca Ferretti, Michael Parker, Michelle Kendall, and David Bonsall. 2020. "Digital Contact Tracing: Comparing the Capabilities of Centralised and Decentralised Data Architectures to Effectively Suppress the COVID-19 Epidemic Whilst Maximising Freedom of Movement and Maintaining Privacy." https://github.com/BDI-pathogens/ covid-19_instant_tracing/blob/master/Centralised%20and%20decentralised%20systems%20for%20contact%20tracing.pdf.

FTC. 2012. "Protecting Consumer Privacy in an Era of Rapid Change." FTC Report. Recommendations for Businesses and Policymakers. Federal Trade Commission. https://www.ftc.gov/sites/default/files/documents/reports/ federal-trade-commission-report-protecting-consumer-privacy- era-rapid-change-recommendations/120326privacyreport.pdf.

———. 2020. "Privacy & Data Security Update: 2019." Federal Trade Commission. https://www.ftc.gov/system/files/documents/reports/privacy-data- security-update-2019/2019-privacy-data-security-report-508.pdf.

Furlanello, Cesare, Stefano Merler, Stefano Menegon, Sebastiano Mancuso, and Gianni Bertiato. 2002. "New WEBGIS Technologies for Geo-Location of

Epidemiological Data: An Application for the Surveillance of the Risk of Lyme Borreliosis Disease." Giornale Italiano Di Aritmologia e Cardiostimolazione, Special Issue Proceedings of the 15th Int. Congress "The New Frontiers of Arrhythmias," 5 (1): 241–45.

Gan, Nectar, and David Culver. 2020. "China Is Fighting the Coronavirus with a Digital QR Code. Here's How It Works." CNN Business. April 16, 2020. https://www.cnn.com/2020/04/15/asia/china-coronavirus-qr-code-intl-hnk/index.html.

Gibson, Dustin G., Adaeze C. Wosu, George William Pariyo, Saifuddin Ahmed, Joseph Ali, Alain B. Labrique, Iqbal Ansary Khan, Elizeus Rutebemberwa, Meerjady Sabrina Flora, and Adnan A. Hyder. 2019. "Effect of Airtime Incentives on Response and Cooperation Rates in Non-Communicable Disease Interactive Voice Response Surveys: Randomised Controlled Trials in Bangladesh and Uganda." BMJ Global Health 4 (5): e001604. https://doi.org/10.1136/bmjgh-2019-001604.

Giglio, Mike. 2020. "Would You Sacrifice Your Privacy to Get Out of Quarantine?" The Atlantic, April 22, 2020. https://www.theatlantic.com/politics/archive/2020/04/coronavirus-pandemic-privacy-civil-liberties-911/609172/.

Guariglia, Matthew. 2020. "The Dangers of COVID-19 Surveillance Proposals to the Future of Protest." Electronic Frontier Foundation. April 29, 2020. https://www.eff.org/deeplinks/2020/04/some-covid-19-surveillance-proposals-could-harm-free-speech-after-covid-19.

Hadavas, Chloe. 2020. "How Effective Are Contact Tracing Apps?" Slate Magazine, May 13, 2020. https://slate.com/technology/2020/05/contact-tracing-apps-less-effective-iceland.html.

Hamilton, Isobel Asher. 2020. "Poland Made an App That Forces Coronavirus Patients to Take Regular Selfies to Prove They're Indoors or Face a Police Visit." Business Insider. March 23, 2020. https://www.businessinsider.com/poland-app-coronavirus-patients-mandaotory-selfie-2020-3.

Hargittai, Eszter, Minh Hao Nguyen, Jaelle Fuchs, Jonathan Gruber, Will Marler, Amanda Hunsaker, and Gökçe Karaoglu. 2020. "Covid-19 Study on Digital Media and the Coronavirus Pandemic." Internet Use and Society Division, Institute of Communication and Media Research, University of Zurich. http://webuse.org/covid/.

Hargittai, Eszter, and Elissa Redmiles. 2020. "Will Americans Be Willing to Install COVID-19 Tracking Apps?" Scientific American Blog Network. April 28, 2020. https://blogs.scientificamerican.com/observations/will-americans-be-willing-to-install-covid-19-tracking-apps/.

Hart, Vi, Divya Siddarth, Bethan Cantrell, Lila Tretikov, Peter Eckersley, John Langford, Scott Leibrand, et al. 2020. "Outpacing the Virus: Digital Response to Containing the Spread of COVID-19 While Mitigating Privacy Risks." Whitepaper 5. COVID-19 Rapid Response Impact Initiative. Edmond J. Safra Center for Ethics. https://drive.google.com/file/d/1vIN2AX-DDNW-SoaHq8xsoRJ2jkR_CckX/view.

Hemming, K., T. P. Haines, P. J. Chilton, A. J. Girling, and R. J. Lilford. 2015. "The Stepped Wedge Cluster Randomised Trial: Rationale, Design, Analysis, and Reporting." BMJ 350 (February). https://doi.org/10.1136/bmj.h391.

Hendrix, Steve, and Ruth Eglash. 2020. "Israel Is Using Cellphone Surveillance to Warn Citizens: You May Already Be Infected." Washington Post. Accessed May 19, 2020. https://www.washingtonpost.com/world/middle_east/israel-is-using-cellphone-surveillance-to-warn-citizens-you-may-already-be-infected/2020/03/19/68267294-69e7-11ea-b199-3a9799c54512_story.html.

Heneghan, Carl, Jon Brassey, and Tom Jefferson. 2020. "COVID-19: What Proportion Are Asymptomatic?" Centre for Evidence-Based Medicine. https://www.cebm.net/covid-19/covid-19-what-proportion-are-asymptomatic/.

HHS. 2019. "Public Health Emergency Declaration." Public Health Emergency. Accessed May 19, 2020. https://www.phe.gov/Preparedness/legal/Pages/phedeclaration.aspx.

Hickey, Matt. 2014. "Carriers Can Now Install Apps On Android Handsets Without Customers' Permission." Forbes. December 1, 2014. https://www.forbes.com/sites/matthickey/2014/12/01/carriers-can-now-install-apps-on-android-handsets-without-customers-permission/.

Hinch, Robert, Will Probert, Anel Nurtay, Michelle Kendall, Chris Wymant, Matthew Hall, Katrina Lythgoe, et al. 2020. "Effective Configurations of a Digital Contact Tracing App: A Report to NHSX." file:///Users/ameliahood/Downloads/Report%20-%20Effective%20App%20Configurations%20(1).pdf.

Ingram, David. 2020. "Apple, Google Push Makers of Coronavirus Apps Not to Record User Location." May 4 2020. NBC News. Accessed May 19, 2020. https://www.nbcnews.com/tech/tech-news/coronavirus-apps-won-t-be-able-record-users-location-apple-n1199586.

Iwaya, Leonardo H., Jane Li, Simone Fischer-Hübner, Rose-Mharie Åhlfeldt, and Leonardo A. Martucci. 2019. "E-Consent for Data Privacy: Consent Management for Mobile Health Technologies in Public Health Surveys and

Disease Surveillance." Studies in Health Technology and Informatics 264 (August): 1223–27. https://doi.org/10.3233/SHTI190421.

"Joint Statement on Contact Tracing." 2020, April 19. https://cryptobriefing. com/wp-content/uploads/2020/04/Joint-Statement-from-Researchers.pdf.

Kahn Gilmor, Daniel. 2020. "Principles for Technology-Assisted Contact-Tracing." White Paper. American Civil Liberties Union. https://www.aclu .org/report/aclu-white-paper-principles-technology-assisted-contact-tracing.

Kim, Max S. 2020. "Seoul's Radical Experiment in Digital Contact Tracing." The New Yorker, April 17, 2020. https://www.newyorker.com/news/ news-desk/seouls-radical-experiment-in-digital-contact-tracing.

Kim, Nemo. 2020. "'More Scary than Coronavirus': South Korea's Health Alerts Expose Private Lives." The Guardian, March 6, 2020, sec. World news. https://www.theguardian.com/world/2020/mar/06/more-scary-than-coronavirus-south-koreas-health-alerts-expose-private-lives.

Kirzinger, Ashley, Liz Hamel, Cailey Muñana, Audrey Kearney, and Mollyann Brodie. 2020. "KFF Health Tracking Poll – Late April 2020: Coronavirus, Social Distancing, and Contact Tracing." Kaiser Family Foundation (blog). April 24, 2020. https://www.kff.org/coronavirus-covid-19/issue-brief/ kff-health-tracking-poll-late-april-2020/.

Knobel, Cory, and Geoffrey C. Bowker. 2011. "Computing Ethics: Value in Design." Communications of the ACM 54 (7): 26–28. https://doi.org/ doi:10.1145/1965724.1965735.

Lee, Ramon, Rosa R. Cui, Kathryn E. Muessig, Harsha Thirumurthy, and Joseph D. Tucker. 2014. "Incentivizing HIV/STI Testing: A Systematic Review of the Literature." AIDS and Behavior 18 (5): 905–12. https:// doi.org/10.1007/s10461-013-0588-8.

Leprince-Ringuet, Daphne. 2020. "Contact-Tracing Apps: Why the NHS Said No to Apple and Google's Plan." ZDNet. April 28, 2020. https://www. zdnet.com/article/contact-tracing-apps-why-the-nhs-said-no-to-apple-and-googles-plan/.

Lovejoy, Ben. 2020. "NHS Contact Tracing App: Hands-on as the Test Goes Live." 9to5Mac (blog). May 7, 2020. https://9to5mac.com/2020/05/07/ nhs-contact-tracing/.

Mahmood, Sultan, Khaled Hasan, Michelle Colder Carras, and Alain Labrique. 2020. "Global Preparedness Against COVID-19: We Must Leverage the Power of Digital Health." JMIR Public Health and Surveillance 6 (2): e18980. https://doi.org/10.2196/18980.

Mathews, Simon C., Michael J. McShea, Casey L. Hanley, Alan Ravitz, Alain B. Labrique, and Adam B. Cohen. 2019. "Digital Health: A Path to

Validation." Npj Digital Medicine 2 (1): 1–9. https://doi.org/10.1038/s41746-019-0111-3.

Mello, By Michelle M., and C. Jason Wang. 2020. "Ethics and Governance for Digital Disease Surveillance." Science, May. https://doi.org/10.1126/science.abb9045.

Mills Rodrigo, Chris. 2020. "Digital Contact Tracing Is Becoming Available, but Is It Effective?" The Hill. May 7, 2020. https://thehill.com/policy/technology/496498-digital-contact-tracing-is-becoming-available-but-is-it-effective.

MIT. n.d. "Private Kit: Safe Paths; Privacy-by-Design Covid19 Solutions Using GPS+Bluetooth for Citizens and Public Health Officials." Safepaths. Accessed May 20, 2020. https://safepaths.mit.edu/.

"Mobile Cellular Subscriptions (per 100 People)." 2018. World Telecommunication/ICT Development Report. International Telecommunication Union. https://data.worldbank.org/indicator/IT.CEL.SETS.P2.

Moore, Sarah, Anne-Marie Tassé, Adrian Thorogood, Ingrid Winship, Ma'n Zawati, and Megan Doerr. 2017. "Consent Processes for Mobile App Mediated Research: Systematic Review." JMIR MHealth and UHealth 5 (8): e126. https://doi.org/10.2196/mhealth.7014.

Morse, Jack. 2020. "North Dakota Launched a Contact-Tracing App. It's Not Going Well." Mashable. Accessed May 19, 2020. https://mashable.com/article/north-dakota-contact-tracing-app/.

Muller, Robert T. 2020. "COVID-19 Brings a Pandemic of Conspiracy Theories." Psychology Today. April 24, 2020. https://www.psychologytoday.com/blog/talking-about-trauma/202004/covid-19-brings-pandemic-conspiracy-theories.

Mulligan, Stephen P., and Chris D. Linebaugh. 2019. "Data Protection Law: An Overview." R45631. Congressional Research Service. https://crsreports.congress.gov/product/pdf/R/R45631.

National Commission for the Protection of Human Subjects of Biomedical and Behavioral Research. 1979. "The Belmont Report: Ethical Principles and Guidelines for the Protection of Human Subjects of Research." US Dept of Health & Human Services, Office of Human Research Protections. https://www.hhs.gov/ohrp/regulations-and-policy/belmont-report/read-the-belmont-report/index.html.

NDDoH. 2020. "North Dakota Launches Care19 App to Combat COVID-19." North Dakota Department of Health. April 7, 2020. https://www.health.nd.gov/news/north-dakota-launches-care19-app-combat-covid-19.

NYC DOH. 2020. "Age-Adjusted Rates of Lab Confirmed COVID-19 Nonhospitalized Cases, Estimated Non-Fatal Hospitalized Cases, and Persons Known to Have Died per 100,000 by Race/Ethnicity Group." New York

City Department of Health. https://www1.nyc.gov/assets/doh/downloads/pdf/imm/covid-19-deaths-race-ethnicity-04242020-1.pdf.

O'Rielly, Michael. 2018. "FCC Regulatory Free Arena." Federal Communications Commission. June 1, 2018. https://www.fcc.gov/news-events/blog/2018/06/01/fcc-regulatory-free-arena.

OSHA. 2020. "Guidance on Preparing Workplaces for COVID-19." OSHA 3990-03 2020. Department of Labor, Occupational Safety and Health Act of 1970. https://www.osha.gov/Publications/OSHA3990.pdf.

Pallmann, Philip, Alun W. Bedding, Babak Choodari-Oskooei, Munyaradzi Dimairo, Laura Flight, Lisa V. Hampson, Jane Holmes, et al. 2018. "Adaptive Designs in Clinical Trials: Why Use Them, and How to Run and Report Them." BMC Medicine 16 (1): 29. https://doi.org/10.1186/s12916-018-1017-7.

Pew Research Center. 2017. "U.S. Muslims Concerned About Their Place in Society, but Continue to Believe in the American Dream." Religion & Public Life. Pew Research Center. https://www.pewforum.org/2017/07/26/findings-from-pew-research-centers-2017-survey-of-us-muslims/.

———. 2020. "Demographics of Mobile Device Ownership and Adoption in the United States." Internet & Technology. Pew Research Center. Accessed May 19, 2020. https://www.pewresearch.org/internet/fact-sheet/mobile/.

PHLS. 2002. "Principles of the Ethical Practice of Public Health." Public Health Leadership Society. https://www.apha.org/-/media/files/pdf/membergroups/ethics/ethics_brochure.ashx.

PIH. 2020a. "Part I: Testing, Contact Tracing and Community Management of COVID-19." PIH Guide | COVID-19. STOP COVID. Partners in Health. https://www.pih.org/sites/default/files/2020-04/PIH_Guide_COVID_Part_I_Testing_Tracing_Community_Managment_4_4.pdf.

———. 2020b. "Box It In." PIH Guide | COVID-19. Partners in Health. https://preventepidemics.org/covid19/resources/box-it-in/.

Resolve to Save Lives. 2020. "COVID-19 Contact Tracing Playbook." Vital Strategies. https://contacttracingplaybook.resolvetosavelives.org/.

Reston, Maeve, Kristina Sgueglia, and Cheri Mossburg. 2020. "Governors on East and West Coasts Form Pacts to Decide When to Reopen Economies." CNN Politics. April 13, 2020. https://www.cnn.com/2020/04/13/politics/states-band-together-reopening-plans/index.html.

Rithalia, Amber, Catriona McDaid, Sara Suekarran, Lindsey Myers, and Amanda Sowden. 2009. "Impact of Presumed Consent for Organ Donation on Donation Rates: A Systematic Review." BMJ 338 (January). https://doi.org/10.1136/bmj.a3162.

Rodrigues, Rafaela, Alina Husain, Amanda Couture-Carron, Leslye E. Orloff, and Nawal H. Ammar. 2018. "Promoting Access to Justice for Immigrant and Limited English Proficient Crime Victims in an Age of Increased Immigration Enforcement: Initial Report from a 2017 National Survey." Washington, DC: National Immigrant Women's Advocacy Project, American University, Washington College of Law. http://niwaplibrary.wcl.american.edu/wp-content/uploads/Immigrant-Access-to-Justice-National-Report.pdf.

Simpson, Erin, and Adam Conner. 2020. "Digital Contact Tracing to Contain the Coronavirus." Center for American Progress. https://www.americanprogress.org/issues/technology-policy/news/2020/04/22/483521/digital-contact-tracing-contain-coronavirus/.

Singer, Eleanor, and Cong Ye. 2013. "The Use and Effects of Incentives in Surveys." The ANNALS of the American Academy of Political and Social Science 645 (1): 112–41. https://doi.org/10.1177/0002716212458082.

Thornton, Rebecca L. 2008. "The Demand for, and Impact of, Learning HIV Status." The American Economic Review 98 (5): 1829–63. https://doi.org/10.1257/aer.98.5.1829.

US DOE. 2009. "State Regulation of Private Schools." US Dept of Education, Office of Non-Public Education. https://www2.ed.gov/admins/comm/choice/regprivschl/regprivschl.pdf.

Valentino-DeVries, Jennifer. 2020. "Cellphone Carriers Face $200 Million Fine for Not Protecting Location Data." The New York Times, February 28, 2020, sec. Technology. https://www.nytimes.com/2020/02/28/technology/fcc-cellphones-location-data-fines.html.

Valentino-DeVries, Jennifer, Natasha Singer, and Aaron Krolik. 2020. "A Scramble for Virus Apps That Do No Harm." The New York Times, April 29, 2020, sec. Business. https://www.nytimes.com/2020/04/29/business/coronavirus-cellphone-apps-contact-tracing.html.

Washington Post–UMD. "Washington Post-University of Maryland National Poll." 2020. Washington Post. April 21, 2020. https://www.washingtonpost.com/context/washington-post-university-of-maryland-national-poll-april-21-26-2020/3583b4e9-66be-4ed6-a457-f6630a550ddf/.

Watson, Crystal, Anita Cicero, James Blumenstock, and Michael Fraser. 2020. "A National Plan to Enable Comprehensive COVID-19 Case Finding and Contact Tracing in the US." Johns Hopkins Bloomberg School of Public Health: Center for Health Security and the Association of State and Territorial Health Officials. https://www.centerforhealthsecurity.org/our-work/pubs_archive/pubs-pdfs/2020/200410-national-plan-to-contact-tracing.pdf.

WHO. 2017. "WHO Guidelines on Ethical Issues in Public Health Surveillance."
World Health Organization. https://www.who.int/ethics/publications/
public-health-surveillance/en/.
———. 2020. "Coronavirus Disease 2019 (COVID-19)." Situation Report 73.
World Health Organization. https://www.who.int/docs/default-source/coro-
naviruse/situation-reports/20200402-sitrep-73-covid-19.pdf.

Lightning Source UK Ltd.
Milton Keynes UK
UKHW022227080620
364668UK00008B/705